Love, labour and loss

STILLBIRTH AND NEONATAL DEATH

**Jo Benson and
Dawn Robinson-Walsh**

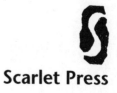

Scarlet Press

Published by Scarlet Press 1996
5 Montague Road, London E8 2HN

British Library Cataloguing-in-Publication Data
A catalogue record for this book is available
from the British Library
ISBN 1 85727 063 0

Designed and produced for Scarlet Press by
Chase Production Services, Chipping Norton, OX7 5QR
Typeset from the authors' disk by
Stanford Desktop Publishing Services, Milton Keynes
Printed in the EC by J.W. Arrowsmith Ltd, Bristol

There is an old adage that
once you have become a parent,
no one can take that away from you.

This book is for parents everywhere
who have known what it is to suffer
the great loss, that of their child.

Contents

Acknowledgements

Our thanks must go to all our contributors who have given us privileged insight into their experiences of loss. Not all the reports we received can be included in this book, for want of space, but that doesn't make those that aren't reproduced any less valuable, and everyone we have heard from can rest assured that their stories have helped to shape the content of this book.

We are indebted to two charities, SANDS (Stillbirth and Neonatal Death Society) and BLISSLINK/NIPPERS (National Information Forum for Parents of Prematures, Education, Resources and Support) for their help in publicising our request for reports and for providing invaluable information. We particularly wish to thank Bridget Yule, Information Officer at SANDS, who has been extremely patient and helpful.

In appreciation of the special help of BLISSLINK/NIPPERS in providing information for the introduction to this book, and to aid the organisation with its work, the charity will receive a donation from the authors.

Thanks to Sara Forrest, midwife, and Ann Mercer of Radcliffe Citizens' Advice Bureau for providing information on complaining about negligent hospital treatment, and to Robert Talbot, a medical negligence solicitor, for checking the legal aspects included in the book. The medical information in chapter 3 has been checked by Derek Tuffnell, consultant obstetrician and gynaecologist at Bradford Royal Infirmary; again, his help has been invaluable. Jenni Thomas has also provided tremendous help and support.

Many thanks also to our editor, the very patient Diana Russell, and to Sue Richards and Hilary Benson for their valued help with proofreading.

Finally, thanks must go to our endlessly patient husbands, Adrian and Andrew, who soothed our brows and lived to tell the tale.

Introduction

This book was inspired when we compiled our first book, a volume on parental experiences of childbirth, *Labours of Love* (1993). We were both (sadly) very much surprised by the number of parents who contacted us, asking us to write a book about losing a baby. Originally, this book was to be just that: a look at parental testimony about losing a child at various stages of pregnancy, during childbirth and in the first year of a child's life. We were not prepared for the overwhelming number of people who wrote to us and kindly sent us their reports in an attempt to help others in a similar situation. It seemed that each type of loss was worthy of a book in itself, and this volume is devoted to the issues of stillbirth and neonatal death.

Today, there is a wealth of information available for pregnant women and their partners about preparation for childbirth, labour and the early months of parenthood. There is still, however, a dearth of information about losing a baby, which is a devastating experience.

Parents who lose a baby before, during or after birth will find the terms 'neonatal', 'perinatal' and 'stillbirth' frequently used. It is helpful to have these defined. A stillborn child is any child born after the twenty-fourth week of pregnancy which did not, at any time after being completely out of its mother's body, breathe or show any other signs of life. Neonatal is a term used to describe a newborn baby – a neonatal death is where the baby is born alive but dies during the first few weeks of life. Perinatal refers to the period between the seventh month of pregnancy and the first week of life, so a baby who is born prematurely and fails to survive is technically classed as a perinatal death.

It has to be acknowledged that not all pregnancies end in the birth of a perfect, healthy baby. Despite the fact that statistics show a steady decline in the numbers of stillbirths and perinatal deaths, there are still thousands of parents in the UK affected annually by the trauma of losing their babies.

Official government statistics for 1991 (the latest available data) show that out of a total of 702,134 births, no less than 3,249 were stillborn. (This does not include neonatal deaths.) These figures can be broken down to show that out of 359,974 male babies there were 1,721 stillbirths, and of 342,160 females a total of 1,528 were stillborn.

The main causes of neonatal death were (by a long way) malformations of the heart and circulatory systems – this was attributed as a principle or underlying cause of 439 such deaths. For stillbirths, the greatest problem was central nervous system malformations, with 61 deaths attributed to this.

In the world of medicine, and in society in general, attitudes to the loss of a child at or shortly after birth have changed significantly during the twentieth century. Although some of our contributors here feel that there is still some distance to travel, we are surely moving in the right direction in terms of our recognition of the heartfelt grief felt by bereaved parents.

Babies have been born dead or died at birth since the dawn of time, and parents have suffered, often in silence. However, where women experience fewer pregnancies and have greater expectations of normal pregnancies, the feelings of loss may be intensified compared with the same event in the days before universally available birth control, when the loss of a baby may have been a time of sadness tinged with relief at not having one more mouth to feed. Not all pregnancies are wanted, and not all parents will feel tremendous loss at a baby's death, but most women who have carried a child to term will have developed some strong feelings and a relationship with their baby. This book is for those who are suffering. It is an attempt to show that their experience is shared, and that the feelings they may have are completely normal and acceptable.

Today, there are three major reasons why a baby may die. These are reduced oxygen supply due to problems with the placenta, known as asphyxia during birth; major physical abnormality which cannot be corrected; or prematurity. In the not so distant past, medical professionals did not have instant access to equipment which could assess oxygen supply and give advance warning of any problems. Intervention is now more likely in childbirth if there is a problem during labour, and many abnormalities may be detected in advance by ultrasound scanning of the baby in the womb.

Some commentators have noted that socio-economic conditions have also played a part in baby deaths. Perinatal deaths tend to be higher in socio-economic groups IV and V (semi-skilled and unskilled manual workers), who have always had and still have differential access to medical care, compared with middle-class groups. In addition, some deaths have been associated with poor foetal growth, which may be linked with drugs, smoking, excess alcohol intake and dietary deficiencies. The reports in this book, however, mainly reflect the many other factors which are involved, most of which are unpredictable.

Janet Palmer, previously of BLISSLINK/NIPPERS, has kindly contributed the following piece about the death of a baby on a neonatal or Special Care Unit. She writes as a professional, but also as someone who has experienced such a devastating loss herself (her personal report is included in chapter 5).

The death of a baby on a neonatal or Special Care Baby Unit (SCBU) is different from any other loss. Not easier, or harder to cope with, but different. It's different from a stillbirth or late miscarriage because the baby is born alive – during labour there is at least some hope. It's different from a cot death because the baby has usually never come home. The time scale is altered as well, especially with premature births. Instead of the sudden shock of stillbirth, miscarriage or cot death, there is the realisation that the baby is going to be born too early. Once the baby is in SCBU, the parents experience a whole range of emotions, ranging from optimism to despair, and the fight for life may last a few brief hours or many weeks or months. The end can come in several ways. It may be sudden and unexpected; a baby making good progress may develop a serious infection such as NEC (necrotising enterocolitis) or meningitis; there may be a slow deterioration in the baby's condition; or the time may come when the doctors suggest that there is little point in continuing and the ventilator is switched off. Not all babies taken to SCBU are born prematurely; some have congenital abnormalities, develop problems during labour or have breathing difficulties at birth. Many sick babies are delivered by Caesarean section, which means it takes the mother longer to recover physically.

While the baby is in SCBU the parents build up a relationship with the baby, but it is an artificial relationship in hospital surroundings. Contact with the baby is often limited. If the parents have other children, it is difficult to spend many hours at the hospital; if the baby is on a ventilator, cuddles are rare treats and physical contact tends to be little more than putting a hand through the portholes to stroke a back or allow a tiny hand to curl round a finger.

Parents get into a routine of visiting the hospital regularly to see their baby, and generally feel close to the doctors and nurses caring for him or her. When the baby dies, not only do they lose their child, but the relationship with the unit is terminated abruptly. They can also feel that their baby has suffered a lot of pain during his or her life, and that they are guilty or responsible for this. They may even wish that treatment had never been given in the first place. Sometimes the parents are relieved when the baby dies, because he or she is no longer suffering. They can also feel guilty about not having spent enough time with the baby, or not having visited often enough, or perhaps angry if they have not been able to see the baby. This can occur, for example, if the mother has had a Caesarean and no one is able to take her to see the baby, or if the baby is transferred to a different hospital.

1 The legacy of loss

There is no death as sad as the death of a child. All bereaved parents experience heartbreak, loneliness and isolation following the death of their child. Thankfully, it is now realised that such parents need comfort, support and encouragement to come to terms with their loss. The Compassionate Friends, a nationwide organisation for bereaved parents, points out that parents need to be helped towards realisation that 'after the pain and turmoil, life will come to have meaning once more'.

In times past (and not so distantly past) childbirth was seen as a precarious business for both mother and child. Many women lost their babies through stillbirth and neonatal death – even if their pregnancies had come to term – in the days before scanning, electronic foetal monitoring and other routine procedures which today help alert staff to a potential problem. Nowadays parents expect childbirth to be safe, and where our grandmothers may have expected to lose a baby at birth or during infancy, the death of a child is now a reversal (in western society at least) of our natural expectations. Parents today feel that with the excellent medical care we have available, screening procedures carried out during pregnancy and intervention to assist delivery if the baby is 'in distress' or in a difficult position such as breech, the outcome of a pregnancy should be a healthy live baby. Sadly, this is still not always the case – perhaps life and death are not predictable enough for it ever to be.

This is an essential chapter because although we wish to concentrate on what is happening to bereaved parents now, rather than dwell on the unsatisfactory procedures of the past, comparisons are well worth making. In researching this book, we came across a number of women who had suffered the stillbirths of their babies many years ago, and whose grieving had been made more difficult and prolonged by the procedures carried out at the time. We include reports from different mothers who lost babies

1

during the period from the 1930s to the late 1970s, whose grief is still very raw and has been inadequately counselled.

The first report comes from a mother who lost twin girls more than 20 years ago. Today, it is highly likely that spina bifida (from which the girls suffered) would have been detected before birth, so the mother would at least have had some preparation for potential problems developing.

The mother's experience occurred in Germany, but the general approach in many hospitals in the UK too was not to let mothers see their stillborn offspring and to pretend that the pregnancy had never occurred, with the mother expected to rally round as if nothing had happened.

Lynda

Some years ago, I gave birth to twin girls; they died just a few minutes after they were born. They both had spina bifida; this I would have accepted and I could have cared for them, but I was told by doctors it was 'for the best'.

I didn't know I was having twins until about one hour before they were born. My husband was in the army, stationed in Germany, and I was out there with him. I had been to see a doctor at the hospital and told him I didn't feel too good. He said I had a murmur on my back – this turned out to be one of the twins' heartbeats.

I was on my own when I started in labour and I had to get myself to my husband's army camp where I could see a doctor. When I told the receptionist that I was 28 weeks pregnant and that my baby was on the way, she told me to sit down and when the doctor had time he would see me.

After ten minutes I knew something was going drastically wrong. I had had two miscarriages before, and a son who is now 24 years old. I asked if I could go into a room on my own and the receptionist reluctantly agreed. A young nurse came in and I told her what was happening and she brought the doctor straight away. He came and examined me and said, 'Oh my God, it's twins and they're on their way.' It was one real mad panic to get me out of the medical centre to the nearest hospital, 20 miles away.

When I got there, nobody could speak English. They started to shave me but couldn't finish as I wanted to push; they then decided to give me an injection to put me to sleep. I woke up covered in blood with nobody there, just a drip in my arm. I shouted for my husband and a nurse came. She said in broken English, 'Your babies have died – they were girls.'

They put me in an ambulance. I searched that ambulance for my babies; the nurse eventually told me she had them in the front with her. I wanted to look at them; they wouldn't let me. I asked what they would do with them. They said they were to be cremated and their ashes would be scattered under a tree in the hospital grounds. I only wish I could have believed this. I begged for those babies but no one listened to me. They put me in a room with a lady who had just had an abortion, told me to pull myself together and gave me some 'nerve' tablets which I gave back to the doctor.

I live with this every day of my life. I wanted to bring my babies back to England. I have no names for them, no birth certificates. I have seen my medical documents this year and it says on them: 'Miscarriage, 28 weeks, twin girls'. Maybe if I had been treated a little better we may have tried again. People say to me, 'Have you any children?' and I reply, 'Yes, I have a son.' They always comment about only one; they do not know the heartbreak inside when they say this to me. I will never forget them; they are with me every day and I will live forever thinking, 'If only'.

It is now recognised that grieving takes a very long time, and that a period of adjustment has to take place. Families need outlets for their emotions. Seeing their dead babies, and holding them, is helpful in allowing the healing process to begin. Some parents today choose not to see their stillborn babies, and later often regret that decision. Frequently, this seems due to the parents' idea that their babies will look somehow monstrous and be abhorrent to them, but this is rarely the case. Having contact with, holding and loving the baby is a first stage of healing, and leaves the parents with at least some memories.

Historic procedures also often meant that the parents were unable to play any part in arranging a funeral for their baby, and were unable therefore to have a service which held religious or symbolic meaning for them, or a burial/cremation place where they could visit. It was as if, to the outside world at least, their baby had never existed.

Many reports we received highlighted the point that people who had experienced stillbirth before the days of explanations and counselling decided not to try for further pregnancies, and many

were further saddened by the lost opportunity to add to their
families.

For some years, there have been charities which have been able
to help with such bereavement. For example, the Compassionate
Friends was founded in 1969, although it was not then a national
organisation. However, the important point is that help and
counselling were not offered at the place where the loss occurred,
in the hospitals. Newly bereaved parents were and are not really
in any state to seek out such information for themselves where
it is not offered as a matter of course. Happily, things are different
today; hospitals often can and do assist by giving information and
leaflets to parents, and by offering to contact an organisation such
as SANDS for them. Many hospitals now also have a quiet room
where parents can be together with their dead or dying baby in
privacy.

One of the many problems affecting bereaved parents has been
(and to some extent still is) related to communication between
hospitals and those working in community medicine. Sometimes
the information about a stillbirth or neonatal death may not
reach the community midwife, GP or health visitor, and it can be
extremely distressing to parents when these people turn up on their
doorstep unaware of the loss which has occurred. However, the
Royal College of Midwives Trust offers assurances that
communication is improving. Bereavement counselling was not
generally considered a part of the work of midwives or doctors in
the past, but this issue is now being addressed. Midwives today
receive more training, and information in this area of interpersonal
skills is constantly updated. When communication systems do
work, as in the majority of cases, the community midwife can be
a great help – midwives are legally obliged to visit women for up
to 28 days following a birth regardless of the outcome, though
most only usually visit for around ten days. In addition,
bereavement counsellors are available in many areas, and hospital
chaplains will usually visit bereaved parents unless requested
not to.

The next report, by Shirley, is an illustration of one occasion
when communications broke down.

Shirley
My son Paul was born in September 1975. I will never know if
it was instinct, but throughout my pregnancy I kept going off
the idea.

In the event, the labour was easy. I went into hospital at 7pm and he was born at 9.10 that evening. They took me to a huge ward and took Paul straight to the nursery. I remember looking at him the next day and thinking he looked blue around the mouth and on the soles of his feet, and he seemed to be panting. The nurses reassured me that it was just that he had been delivered so quickly.

It was the next day before doctors discovered serious heart problems – his heart was enlarged. They transferred him to a London hospital, but left me behind. Before he left they gave him a rapid baptism, getting me out of the bath to do it and allowing no time for my husband to join us. There was no question of transferring me until I had been discharged from maternity, and the staff made no real attempts to communicate with London to find out his progress. Finally, I moved to the mothers' unit at London for three and a half weeks. Paul had a hole in the heart. At five weeks they performed a catheterisation, and then they operated in an attempt to help, but still he died at six and a half weeks.

The local support systems were appalling. The health visitor had not been informed of Paul's death, and I don't think the GP knew either. We were offered absolutely no support. I think the hardest thing was waiting to get pregnant again, which took several months. When finally we conceived, we visited the Genetic Counselling Office in Great Ormond Street, but they reassured me that the chances of a repeat incident were so slim as to be negligible. We subsequently safely delivered Danika, our daughter, and then a son, Peter.

Throughout all my difficulties, I could not have coped without the support of my next-door neighbour. My sister was also a great help – she had also lost a daughter, her first child too, of cot death at one month old.

I feel that one of the very few positive things to come out of all my upset was that I joined Action Research, which funds medical research, in the hope that I can help to prevent other parents from suffering as I did.

The following report in many ways speaks for itself. It involves the loss of a twin. This is a difficult loss to bear, made more so by the fact that many people assume the parents still feel lucky to have one child. But a remaining twin can be a constant reminder of the death of the other. (There is more about this in chapter 2.)

In this report, Janet, highlights the problems she had not only with medical staff but also with the church, when her husband tried to arrange a burial for their child. Fortunately, again, procedures have changed, and medical staff and the clergy now have better training to deal with such situations.

Janet
In 1955, when I was 24 years old, I was delighted to find myself pregnant. At about 16 weeks the doctors decided that I was too big for my dates and I was therefore X-rayed (they did, in those days). This proved that my dates were correct but that I was having twins. As I grew, so did the problem.

Eventually I developed toxaemia and had to be admitted for total bed rest and a salt-free diet. The consultant only turned up on a Wednesday; the rest of the time the medical cover was provided by a houseman doing his six months obstetrics and knowing less than the midwives.

At last it was decided to induce the birth as it was almost full term anyway. I went into labour. Most of the time you were left alone, no husbands or other relatives in those days. In the delivery room were the midwife and various other people who were there to observe a twin delivery, including the houseman. No senior doctor, no paediatrician.

About seven hours from the breaking of the waters my first son was born. He weighed 7lb 7oz (3.4kg), and cried well. Twenty minutes later my second son was born, the same size as his brother, but he did not cry. I was aware of agitation, injections, suckers, but I could not see very well. I could just see that they were holding him upside down and doing something to him.

'I'm afraid you only have the one baby', was all that was said. The third stage of labour had to be got through, and all the usual practical things following a birth. I was exhausted and numb. After that one sentence NOBODY mentioned the dead baby. My husband was told that he only had one baby and that they wished to perform a post-mortem.

At feeding times I was given Christopher to feed and all the nurses said he was a lovely baby. Certainly he was, so why was I so upset? My feelings were in total chaos. What had gone wrong? How come there were two babies yesterday and only one today?

Nobody mentioned my loss, but there was enough milk for two so I was producing milk for the premature babies as well as my own son. The post-mortem was performed and the doctor spoke to my husband (not me). The baby had suffered a tentorial tear – as he was the second twin, he had been propelled rapidly from the top of the uterus to the vagina and there had not been time for the head to be moulded slowly as it went through the birth canal. This had caused the two sides of the head to be compressed together and caused a brain haemorrhage. My husband was told to register the stillbirth as well as the live birth and asked what he wanted done with the baby's body. He asked what was the usual procedure and was told that they usually handed them to an undertaker in a cardboard box to be interred in any convenient grave that happened to be available. We would not know where.

We were both horrified. We decided we wanted the baby to be buried properly in the village churchyard. As the baby had not been baptised, the normal service could not be used, nor could he be taken into the church. As a compromise he could be buried at the side of the churchyard under the trees, but there could be no headstone to mark the place. My husband arranged for a little coffin to be made, collected the baby from the mortuary, took the coffin in his car to the church and was met there by the rector. On a cold January day they said prayers for the baby and buried him.

The whole thing was traumatic for my husband, who had been looking forward to our twins just as much as I was. I came home from hospital with Christopher to two sets of baby clothes, two carry-cots, etc. It started to snow and it was some time before I could go to church to see the little mound in the earth covering our much-wanted baby. There were still the unanswered questions. How could the midwives and doctors let this happen? Why would no one speak to me about it? Why was the church so set in its procedures that it could not let our baby into church simply because he had not been baptised? I deeply regret not having held my son, but am happy that we insisted on a proper burial in a known place.

I felt cheated. I had gone through so much to get my babies. I was still underweight. I was overprotective of my surviving baby and had a constant fear that he too could be taken away from me by some unexpected mishap.

I have never stopped minding. My next two children were born at home. Both were complicated, but I had a feeling that I was in charge at home and that all would be well as long as I kept away from the hospital.

Happily, many things have changed. Parents can hold their stillborn babies and even have photographs taken. Nurses are better trained and taught to understand grief. The attitude of the church has changed. My son's name is entered in a book of remembrance at the church. When my husband died three years ago, our baby's name was added to his headstone. Somehow this proves he existed.

The next report shows the unsympathetic approach of some staff in times past, and also the dangers which mothers often encountered in their attempt to have children. This mother was able to look at her childbearing years positively in retrospect, as she later had healthy pregnancies, but she has obviously never forgotten what happened or how she was treated.

Doris
My first pregnancy was confirmed in May 1938 and from then until three days before the birth, I had no medical attention whatsoever. It was a miserable pregnancy, plagued by morning sickness and resulting depression. My first signs of labour began on Sunday 10 December, but it was not until the following Thursday that the midwife came. She was not unduly concerned and let me continue until Saturday 16 December, when she decided that a doctor had better come. I was given ether, and my baby was eventually delivered with her cord and her little hands around her neck. My husband was downstairs when the doctor came down carrying our baby in his arms. He turned to my husband and said: 'Here is your baby, but she is dead.' His exact words. I was very ill for three weeks after the birth, and my husband was also ill, so my mother came to look after us. There was no one to counsel us, or help in any way. We just had to struggle with our grief and help one another.

I have had five normal pregnancies since, but the birth of our first little daughter remains a very vivid memory.

The following report is a hopeful one. Christine lost her baby daughter 22 years ago. She only sought help three years ago. Again, her experience at the time was awful. The birth was long and hard, the hospital dealt with the burial of the baby and Christine was not allowed to touch her or to hold her. Today's excellent practices of taking photographs of the baby for the parents or keeping locks of his or her hair just did not occur then.

Christine
Rebecca was stillborn on our fourth wedding anniversary and would now be 22 years old. The birth was awful; our daughter had been dead for two weeks and my labour lasted for several days.

When I eventually went home from the hospital, no one talked about Rebecca; it was as if she hadn't existed. I just tried to carry on with my life looking after our two-year-old son. My husband was marvellous; only HE understood, but I bottled all my feelings up for years. We had another son; we loved both our sons, but silently I yearned for my daughter. I had never seen her or touched her – she was just taken away; I didn't know where. If only I had a photograph or a lock of hair – but 20 years ago that didn't happen.

Three years ago, I really began to feel low. My sons were grown up and I longed for my daughter; we would have been going shopping together, choosing clothes together, all the things that mothers and daughters do. Then a friend mentioned SANDS to me. My husband telephoned the number and I was sent information and contact numbers. We were so impressed that last year for our Silver Wedding celebrations, we asked friends to give donations to the society as Rebecca would have been 21 that day. I then decided I would join a group and spoke to a local contact.

She asked if I knew where my daughter was buried, and within two days she had found her. The first time we went to the cemetery it was very emotional, but now we go there every month and recently have put a marble pot where she is buried. Nothing will alter our feelings and we will never forget, but at least now we know where she is. My husband and I are both now contacts for SANDS – we can never thank them enough.

Even so many years on, Christine found that the group she contacted, SANDS, was helpful in assisting with the grief that had been hidden away for so long. In a very practical way, SANDS was able to trace the burial place of her daughter and therefore to help provide a focus for the parents' grieving. SANDS was also able to offer 'befriending' from someone who had experienced a similar loss.

The overwhelming message which comes across from these reports is that while the past treatment of newly bereaved parents was appalling, partly due to little understanding of the grieving process and partly due to patient care which was more orientated to hospital routine than parental needs, there is still time to help parents who lost their babies many years ago. While perhaps nothing can prepare us for suddenly losing a much-wanted baby, there are ways of helping each other through the aftermath. There may not be tangible things which can be done in every case, such as finding out where the baby is buried. But just knowing that others have some idea of how you are affected as a grieving parent, feeling as if all hopes have been lost, is a great help to many people. It can take many years to come to terms with grief, but the process is usually helped along by talking to someone who will listen, who has been through a similar loss, who has empathy and understanding of the feelings which have developed over the years.

While many people can and do manage their grief on their own, in their own way, and feel they do not need outside help, there are surely an equal number who feel the need to resolve their emotions with some extra assistance. For those who can cope alone, perhaps because they have excellent support networks in the shape of family and friends, bereavement and befriending groups are perhaps redundant, but for many people living in a geographically mobile society, with close family and friends at quite a distance, such groups provide an invaluable service.

Sometimes joining such groups, or indeed becoming a befriender, many years after a loss may trigger buried grief which parents thought they had come to terms with. This does not necessarily have to be a problem; it may even enable women who received little help and counselling in the past to be assisted today. Similarly, other losses, such as miscarriage, may bring back old feelings.

One problem which is only touched upon here, but covered in more detail in chapter 7, is the tremendous potential which losing a child has for damaging a marriage and existing family life. People often grieve in different ways and at varying rates which partners may find difficult to deal with. In the following extract, the writer and her husband separated the year following the death of their baby daughter.

Margaret

My first baby, a girl, was born 17 years ago. There were no tests or scans, so it was not picked up that there was anything wrong with her. She was born at 39 weeks after a difficult labour. The staff seemed upset and rushed off with my baby. I caught sight of her for a second before they went and she looked fine to me. I was left alone for about 15 minutes – completely stunned – knowing something was wrong. A nurse came back, asked for a name and told me my baby was going to die so they were christening her. My husband left the hospital very distressed. I never saw my baby again – I began to question whether there ever had been a baby inside me. In the hospital, and once back at home, people discouraged me from crying and seemed to want to pretend it had never happened.

I spent 15 years 'pretending it had never happened'. I often wondered what they had done with my baby. Sometimes I imagined they may have burnt her body at the hospital. A sequence of events then triggered my buried grief: I started befriending newly bereaved parents for SANDS, I had a miscarriage which brought back all the old feelings of loss, and my youngest daughter was born six weeks prematurely and spent three weeks in Special Care. I became very depressed and felt my pain and sadness as if my baby had just died recently. This was the most difficult time for me. I have now recommenced doing befriending work for SANDS, and sometimes talk at hospitals to doctors and midwives. I am currently doing voluntary bereavement counselling.

My baby was not normal, and the situation was handled badly. I was given wrong information, and only found out the facts when I sent for her death certificate recently. I have now found her grave and visit it sometimes and look after it. My husband and I separated the following year, two weeks after the birth of my next baby. I have learnt so much from my experience and I now want to help others to come to terms with their loss.

A Child Bereavement Trust leaflet states that 'grief that is ignored can harm us in countless ways'. It is therefore important to support families during such difficult times, to minimise the long-term psychological consequences. The number of letters we received from people who were still suffering from a lack of recognition of their losses on the part of professionals and those closest to them bears testimony to the fact that treatment at the time of loss plays a vital part in coming to terms with grief.

Even today, while parents may receive better treatment from hospital and community health staff than used to be the case, it may be forgotten that for every death of a baby there are – in addition to grieving parents – grandparents and siblings to consider too. Friends, neighbours and in some cases whole communities may also be affected by the event.

Has it all changed now?

Losing a baby still engenders the same feelings within us, but it may be helpful for parents to know what sort of support they may reasonably expect from medical sources today. Some parents in later reports in this book found it insensitive that they were discharged soon after the birth, or that the private 'couple's rooms' provided were in many cases adjacent to the maternity ward. One hospital offered some helpful comments on this. It pointed out that many women wish to go home as soon as possible after the delivery, and that should be their choice. As for being situated close to maternity wards:

> Women prefer to be nursed by midwives and to be near the maternity ward as they have had a baby, and therefore would not want to feel they had been rejected by the professionals who had looked after them during their pregnancy. Many bereaved women have had obstetric complications and therefore need midwifery care. Many midwives now adopt the approach of family/centred care and support is usually needed for the whole family. Community midwives will visit for as long as required, sometimes several weeks. They act as a point of liaison between the home and hospital consultants, and can talk with the family about fears and anxieties and future pregnancies.

Medical staff today, while still not specifically trained to work with bereaved parents, are able to and frequently do give more time to the mother, providing additional monitoring and discussion about the delivery and timing of the birth. Usually extra care is offered to women who have a history of stillbirth and neonatal loss, as their anxieties are obviously likely to be particularly acute. In such cases the GP – whose approach is often very important to the mother – usually refers the woman to a specialist immediately a pregnancy is diagnosed and obstetricians generally arrange to see such a mother more frequently. Genetic screening may be available and offered if appropriate, and pre-conception counselling may be an option in some areas.

Bereaved parents are usually offered a visit by the hospital chaplain. This is worth considering – these days, chaplains will usually work with parents of any denomination, or indeed of no religious belief, and their role is one of listening and counselling. They may also be able to assist with questions of funeral arrangements.

For helpful voluntary organisations, please refer to Chapter 8.

2 Stillbirth and neonatal death today

Chapter 1 referred to experiences of loss faced by parents some 20–60 years ago. There is no doubt but that, with the passing of time and today's greater knowledge of the importance of bereavement counselling, the losses suffered by these women all those years ago would today be treated with greater compassion and understanding.

It is evident from the data collected in compiling this book that each region, indeed each hospital, has a different level of care for the bereaved. There is no doubt that the medical profession is a caring one, and at the end of the day the treatment parents receive after the traumatic loss of their baby will depend to a great extent on the spirit and sensitivity of the doctors and nurses involved.

There is such intense pain involved in the aftermath of a baby's death that it is hard to believe the attitude of the medical staff can make much difference, yet the message comes across time and time again that gentle words from a nurse or the supporting touch of a doctor's hand have been of immense help. Their advice (sensitively offered) often appears to have been that parents will benefit in the long term from spending time with their baby after his or her death, expressing their love and saying a sad farewell. Without exception, the parents who acted upon such advice were eventually grateful for it.

The attitudes of friends, relatives and neighbours of the bereaved are also crucial. The needs of the sufferers inevitably vary, but in almost every case parents feel hurt when they are not allowed to talk of their loss, and feel shunned and betrayed when others try to pretend that their lost baby never existed. The work of the befrienders from the SANDS organisation has been praised time and time again. Many contributors to this volume have taken comfort from the fact that they have eventually been able to use their pain positively to help others, in some instances by becoming a befriender themselves. Karen is one of these.

Karen
I decided to start a SANDS group because when I lost my baby girl, Gemma, there did not seem to be any help around. My group has now been running for three years; thankfully, I do not get many mums attending but when I can help I try.

For me, my story began eight years ago in June. In the early hours of the morning I awoke with very slight pains. Later I had a show of blood. The pains became quicker. My husband phoned the hospital and I went in at about 6.30am. My labour slowly progressed through the day. A nurse came in and asked me to sign a form, just in case I was torn, so they could stitch me. I remember her very well; she was quite rude, as if I was putting her out.

As the day went on, I progressed into my late stage. The baby's head was visible; 'Keep pushing,' the sister said. It seemed to go on forever. I was given pethidine twice as I was in so much pain. By 9 o'clock I was exhausted.

One nurse was checking the baby's heartbeat with a hand monitor. Suddenly, I could see lots of staff around me. One doctor put his head round the door. The next thing I knew, I was rushed to the forceps room, where my beautiful baby daughter was swiftly glided out of my body. My husband was in tears; I couldn't understand what was going on. Gemma was put on a respirator. Her heart had already stopped when she was inside me. The staff managed to revive her and she was put in an incubator.

I was told that Gemma had got into distress during the birth and her heart stopped for one minute. Gemma managed to live for 16 days on a drip feed; her brain was damaged due to lack of oxygen.

We had Gemma buried in the local cemetery. We were all shattered by what had happened. My mother believes that I was left too long in labour. Even now, I think back and often sit down and cry. I look at her photos and try to imagine how she would look now. Gemma was a big baby, as I went full-term with her.

I went on to have a perfectly healthy girl a year later and then a boy followed.

The next report is a rare contribution from a man. Obviously, men do suffer a great deal from the deaths of their babies, but perhaps fewer feel able to express it in the same way as women.

Likewise, we have had few, if any, contributions from teenagers, although the statistics available demonstrate that there is a higher proportion of stillbirths among mothers who are less than 20 years of age, as Table 1 demonstrates:

Table 1   Stillbirths in England and Wales, 1991 (by age of mother)

	Mother less than 20	Mother more than 20
Live births	42,007	622,230
Stillbirths	292	3,524
Stillbirths per		
1,000 live births	6.95	5.66

Note: These figures do not include perinatal mortality rates (stillbirths plus deaths in the first week of life).
Source: Office of Population Censuses and Surveys, *Infant and Perinatal Mortality*, 1994.

John's contribution shows that his attitude towards the medical services is mixed, and he clearly did not find the comfort outside the hospital that he badly needed.

John
We started IVF treatment in April 1988, after a couple of years of infertility treatment by tablets and normal attempts to become pregnant. Pauline became pregnant first time. Everything was going well until a scan indicated a black mass in the bladder area, interpreted as a sign of a full bladder. Two months later a further scan again indicated a black mass, which on this occasion required further investigation. More scans and tests followed at different hospitals. They indicated that when the baby was born, he might have a problem with his bladder but that it would not be life-threatening.

A urologist first told us of what could be done, but later indicated that due to the cost of treatment the baby would be considered to be outside the city catchment area as far as new medical techniques were concerned. Pauline went to antenatal clinics at two hospitals.

She was admitted to hospital and the baby was born by Caesarean section on 31 January. When I arrived, she was in the recovery ward and the baby was in intensive care. I went to see Pauline and then the doctor broke the news to me that the baby was very seriously ill and could not be moved or operated upon. We were prepared for bad news, but I was absolutely shattered when I became aware of the reality of the situation. Pauline was still very drugged up and she went to see the baby in intensive care in the knowledge that he had been able to pass water. Previously, we had been told in very simple terms that if he could pass water he would be well, given time. Even in the intensive care area, he looked a lovely, well-formed little boy.

The hospital staff could not have been more helpful. The surgeon came and explained that our baby was very seriously ill. The little boy would not survive an operation and he had made the decision for us to allow the baby to die with dignity. I broke down and wept. Poor Pauline was still in a daze and not fully aware of what we had been told.

The surgeon said the baby could be taken out of the incubator and left under the care of the nurses or brought up to the ward for us to look after. We both cuddled and hugged him, hoping that mistakes had been made.

The hospital chaplain came to our room and a christening service was undertaken. We named our son Thomas Anthony Lawrence. He was a beautiful little baby, so marvellously formed on the outside. However, the doctors told us that his whole little body on the inside was damaged, with very few organs not affected. We spent all our time cuddling Thomas and hoping that he was not suffering or hungry. On occasions, his beautiful little face almost went blue as he strove to hold on to life.

Our thoughts at this time were just to make life as comfortable as possible for Thomas. We both felt trapped in a strange world. Thomas kept fighting for his little life and was occasionally sick, but he seemed determined to try to live. I was totally mixed up in my feelings, as I wanted to have Thomas for as long as we could, but at the same time did not want him to suffer unnecessarily. We held Thomas as close to us as we could or held his tiny hands as he lay in his little cot. The nursing staff offered to take him back to the intensive care area at about midnight, but we wanted him to live out his short life in our company.

At about 5am we noticed that Thomas had become very still. The sister took Thomas away and spent some time observing him before coming to confirm that out little son had died. It was inevitable but still a devastating shock. The first feelings I had were of intense bitterness. I was very annoyed by the circumstances which had allowed us to go through such a long period of worry and concern and resulted in our little boy having such a short life.

A post-mortem was carried out and it was discovered that Thomas had been born with a large number of complicated problems, and that his kidneys were so badly damaged they would not have been able to sustain life.

I had to go and register the birth of Thomas and at the same time, his death. I felt I was going through the motions and looked around at all the other parents notifying the births of their children. The registrar assured me that many people had to undergo this terrible experience. It was no real comfort.

We had a very quiet funeral for Thomas. The vicar had married us five years earlier and gave a very appropriate service. We now had to return to our normal life, if anything was going to be normal again. I was going back to work and Pauline's parents came back with us to try to ease her back into the way of life. People at work ignored the subject or avoided me and I wanted to talk about things. People would talk about their families and it would hurt very much. We have never got back to normal and part of our hearts have a space for Thomas.

We have been lucky to adopt a little boy from Romania called Alexei. He has been made aware of his brother and, like us, will grow up never to forget his big brother.

Additional insight into how men respond to the deaths of their babies was provided during an interview with Martin. He and his wife, Vivienne, had a stillborn baby daughter, Kieran. She died in the womb during early labour. Photographs show Kieran to have been a beautiful baby who was a good weight (over 8lb) at birth. A post-mortem found no cause for her death.

Martin, despite his obvious sorrow about the event and love for Kieran, managed to be philosophical:

It's what I call the X-factor. The medics don't know everything. They're human; we're human. We cannot blame the hospital.

There were signs of distress because meconium [see Glossary] was present, but that didn't cause Kieran's death.

Martin cried at the delivery.

I felt sorry for the midwife when she couldn't pick up the heartbeat. I saw her face and thought, 'Oh, no.' Then the doctor came in, and there was talk about position and vernix. Everything had been going so well for us, then it felt as if our legs had been kicked right from underneath us. If we could cope with this, we could cope with anything.

After Kieran's birth, Martin found that the people he worked with treated him differently, as if any display of temper or annoyance at work was because of his and Vivienne's loss. They also tended to ask him how his wife was, never how he was – the assumption was that Vivienne was affected more, or that if they asked Martin how he was, they might be unable to cope with what followed.

After the initial deep grief and shock, Martin found it essential to develop a way of living again.

I put the brakes on and only allowed myself to think of certain things at certain times. This was my strategy for coping. From isolation comes strength; you're on your own, it's make or break, which brings out the best in people. Too much support from others might have meant that our grieving would have been perpetuated. If we were to crack up, it would have put the blame on Kieran. She was perfect; she did nothing wrong. Our behaviour is a reflection of her, and I am not prepared to put the responsibility on to her.

The next contributor is not alone in telling of mixed treatment from hospital staff. After a miscarriage, her next child was stillborn. She describes the registrar and most of the nursing staff as being 'totally embarrassed'. Clearly, doctors and nurses are only human and the overriding impression is that they are not all coached in human compassion and the relevant skills to help suffering parents. At the same time, Jean has much praise for the nurse who kindly kept the body of Jean's daughter in her office overnight: she 'kept her eye on her'. It is clear that such kindness meant much to Jean in her time of great need.

Jean

After having had two sons, both of whom had been born with the cord around their necks but had suffered no lasting ill effects, in August 1990 I found I was pregnant and after the initial shock was very pleased.

On 31 October I went along to the hospital. For my first scan, I drank the necessary pint of water. While I was having the scan, I was asked how many weeks I was and I replied, 'Twelve.' The radiologist told me I needed to drink more water for her to be able to see better. I felt myself go cold; something wasn't right. A midwife came in and they tried again. Everything was quiet and they asked if I had someone with me. They told me they were very sorry but they couldn't find a heartbeat; my baby had died. I was numb. I tried to ring my husband Andy, then my parents; no one was home. I needed to be with Andy; I forced myself to be calm and persuaded the midwife I could drive myself home and she let me go. I got home safely, but God only knows how. Andy was in and I told him what had happened, then collapsed into tears. Andy had to cope with everything, telling family and friends and, worst of all, telling our boys; they were so disappointed. I spent the next day in a daze. I returned to the hospital and they told me I could have a D&C the next morning.

I was put on a side ward, for which I was very grateful, and told I would be examined by a doctor. He announced that my 'abortion' would soon be over and I would be back to normal. The nurse must have seen my distress, and after the doctor left explained that 'abortion' was only a medical term; this didn't make me feel any better. I feel the staff should have been more sensitive to my feelings. Later, after Andy left, I became very upset again. I was told I should pull myself together and think of my boys, but I *was* thinking of them and this added to my distress. I knew what I'd lost. The D&C went well and I left hospital physically fine. My emotional state took longer to heal but I knew now I wanted a baby.

In May 1991 I found I was expecting again and we were delighted. Andy went with me for the first scan. I could hardly get the necessary water down but I needn't have worried – our baby was fine and due on New Year's Eve. I settled into my pregnancy and took good care of myself. Everything was lovely, but then in November, when I was 34 weeks pregnant, my baby became very quiet. I remembered this as quite normal with my boys. On Sunday 10th November I didn't feel her move at all. I spent Monday prodding my stomach; on Tuesday I rang my GP. She told me to go straight to hospital. I was very worried I was going to waste their valuable time. My sister came with me. When we arrived, the midwife put me on to a monitor to trace the baby's heartbeat. The midwife told me that babies normally start to move on the monitor, and she did, one large kick. But I didn't know it was her last. The midwife came back and sent me for a scan. I was quite nervous. I didn't like scan rooms and I still wasn't convinced all was well.

Once more I was on the scan bed. I was asked questions; the lady doing it seemed very nervous. The midwife next to me had removed her glasses. Something was wrong. Was the baby deformed, mentally retarded, Down's syndrome? – it didn't matter, I'd cope with anything. They told me they wanted me to speak to a doctor. There were tears in their eyes when I asked what was wrong. 'I'm so sorry, your baby's died.' I felt like screaming. Why, oh why had I not come in earlier? My sister came in. I could feel the tears falling and could hear myself repeating, 'Not again, please not again.' My sister shouted at me to be calm and I could hear her telling the staff to do a section, that my baby had been alive minutes before. I felt like I was in a bubble. I could hear the conversation but couldn't join in; they were trying to explain it was too late for a section.

Again, I was put on a side ward. I remember a nurse saying I would see a doctor very soon, but all I could think of was the labour; I couldn't go through it, not for a dead baby. Next thing I knew, Andy was there; we held each other and cried.

Two and a half hours later a doctor arrived – not my doctor, just a stranger. He tried to say he was sorry and explained I would be induced the next day. I knew I had to go home and tell our boys what had happened – only the week before I'd promised my eldest son everything would be OK this time. I'd failed. It was the hardest thing I ever did but I wanted to do it myself; I owed them that much. Their reaction was terrible. 'You promised it would be OK,' said my eldest and it ripped my heart in two. I couldn't cope and my parents came to take the boys home with them.

I don't remember much about that night. I didn't sleep, we just cried and held each other.

The next day Andy and I arrived at the hospital and I was asked whether I wanted to stay on maternity or gynaecology.

I didn't know; I didn't care. I was put in a side ward on maternity, but they should have put me away from other babies. Andy and I were left alone for an hour, then my consultant's registrar arrived to explain what was going to happen to me. Why hadn't my consultant come? Was this awful thing that had happened to us not enough to warrant her attention? But I kept quiet and didn't make a fuss. The registrar was totally embarrassed dealing with me, as were most of the nursing staff. I do remember two wonderful midwives, but on the whole I felt very let down.

They started me off with pessaries which put me into slow labour, but I didn't progress much. The day was a painful round of tears and silences, broken by the hospital social worker explaining about death certificates, registering the baby's birth and death, hospital funerals. I did say I wanted a private funeral – I wanted her to have the best; this was the only thing I could do for her.

One midwife who was on duty that day was marvellous with us both. She was an older lady and she gently bullied us into eating and drinking. At the end of the day, the registrar returned and wanted to put me on a drip, but the midwife persuaded her that I was emotionally done in and could take no more.

I remember waking in the night to be greeted by a pregnant nurse asking if I needed to talk. I felt like I'd been slapped in the face but I tried to stay calm and declined her offer. Next morning our nice midwife was on duty and she put me on a drip. Andy arrived. During the day, the dosage of the drip was increased and I was soon in labour. Andy did everything for me: took me to the toilet, helped me soak in a hot bath for the pain and refused to let the nurses help me. By 6 o'clock I needed something to cope with the pain and I was given morphine. I couldn't have an epidural because it wasn't the right day.

We were transferred to the labour unit at 7 o'clock. The next two hours I find very difficult to remember, but Andy told me he felt totally abandoned with me. All that changed with a new midwife, who was the first person to talk about our baby, not 'it'. She talked to us about holding our baby, taking photos, etc. At 9.40pm on 14 November, our daughter Rachel Marie was born at 4lb 7oz (2.02kg) with the cord around her neck, which the midwife gave as the reason for her death, so I decided against a post-mortem, a decision I now regret as every doctor I've spoken to since has seen this as an unlikely cause of death. Having said that, the baby suffered enough in her short life and I didn't want her to go through any more.

My initial reaction after her birth was relief that the physical pain was over and then sheer terror. I couldn't look at my baby. The midwife asked a nurse to take Rachel and wash her and put her in the clothes I'd brought, then sat and talked to us and held me while I cried, and told us how beautiful Rachel was, how perfect, and how she was like a sleeping baby. I pulled myself together and they brought Rachel back; she was perfect, not a mark on her. I needed to hold her and all the love I'd felt when my sons were born was there again for Rachel. I was proud she was so beautiful, with masses of dark hair. She broke my heart; she was the image of her daddy.

Andy had warned me he wouldn't be able to hold her but as soon as he saw her he fell in love with her too and had no difficulty holding her and talking to her. We took a lot of photos and she stayed with us until 1 o'clock in the morning – we have some lovely memories of this time together. I do now regret our boys didn't meet her, although they saw her photo.

Now totally exhausted, I fell asleep and when I awoke I was back on maternity. The midwife told me she'd kept Rachel in her office overnight and kept her eye on her. I will never be able to explain how much this small thing means to me; someone had treated my baby as a baby. The staff on maternity couldn't seem to be rid of me fast enough. We were given her birth and death certificates and told that we could see Rachel again if we needed.

The walk out of the hospital is engraved on my mind; the long corridors with no midwife carrying our healthy baby. We saw Rachel twice more, once at the hospital where we took one more photo and once at the chapel of rest. Rachel was buried on 22 November with a little teddy we had bought when I was expecting her.

The weeks after Rachel's death were extremely hard. Some people came to see us; others avoided us; some even crossed the road to avoid us. I tried not to be hurt by this and by unfortunate remarks made, but some days I was very angry and bitter towards people. I went through quite a range of emotions, from complete despair to thankfulness that this experience had changed Andy and me into less selfish people.

When we returned to hospital to discuss what had happened with my consultant, we had to wait in the maternity waiting room full of expectant mums for 40 minutes. Our consultant told us there was no way we could be sure that the cord was the answer and that two out of four children wasn't bad. I felt sick, and Andy said if she'd been a man he would have hit her.

Gradually, with the help of our families and true friends we are learning to live with our loss, but we'll never forget Rachel. Even now I find the 14th of the month very hard, and special occasions are harder because she's not there.

We do now have a new life in our family to celebrate. Ten weeks after Rachel died, I found I was expecting again and after a very long pregnancy with a lot of worry and upset (this time at a different hospital), our son, Daniel Andrew, was born, being induced at 38 weeks for my sanity.

We love Daniel with all our hearts and he is bringing a lot of happiness back into our lives, but he isn't a replacement for Rachel; he's a person in his own right, as was Rachel.

The problems of those who have had multiple births and lost one or more babies, while one or more survive, deserve separate consideration. The emotions are so mixed. Special help is needed for these people. TAMBA offers a bereavement support group which consists of parents who themselves have lost one or both twins (see chapter 8 for contact details).

A twin pregnancy does carry increased risks of miscarriage, of premature birth with its possible complications, of placental breakdown (which may lead one or both babies to die in the womb), of congenital abnormality and of complications during delivery.

This does not make the loss of a twin any easier. The death of a baby is always a tragic event. What people sometimes fail to realise is that this is not in any way lessened because there happens to be another baby of the same age who has survived. If a woman lost a baby and had a healthy two-year-old, no one would expect her not to grieve for the baby because she also had a toddler. People do tend to make thoughtless remarks, such as: 'How lucky that you have another baby,' or 'Two would have been a handful.' They are trying to be sympathetic and to look for something positive to focus on, but of course it doesn't seem like that to the bereaved parent.

People generally find the death of a baby difficult to talk about. It is easy to avoid the subject with twins because there may be one new baby to admire and it is easier to focus on the positive aspects of the birth. However, the live baby will be a living memory of the lost child for the parents and some may even resent the fact that one baby survived, whereas the other died. Equally, the loss of one baby may make parents unduly anxious about the health of the surviving twin.

TAMBA makes the interesting point that some people feel terribly let down because, as parents expecting twins, they have been considered special, a focus of admiration. Suddenly, all that is gone.

It can be very difficult for a mother to distinguish in her mind between her live baby and her stillborn one. This is where hospital photographs of the dead child can be particularly useful – to help the mother recognise that the baby who died was indeed real. Giving the dead baby a name is also vital. Counselling and other help from health visitors, midwives and GPs can be enormously beneficial. Special care should be taken to ensure that these parents are allowed to grieve, because when two babies are anticipated to have only one is not the consolation that some people believe. Parents in this situation may feel let down. Any lost baby, whether a single child, a twin or triplet, is not replaceable by another.

Statistics show that losing a baby often happens to relatively young parents, so this may be their first experience of personal tragedy. Many will not yet have lost their own parents, or even grandparents, so will not have suffered close loss before. They may also be geographically isolated from their relatives, which may mean that the support they are given by their families will inevitably be limited.

Our next contributor has had more than her share of worries, but is still brave enough to share her emotions with us. We can all, as friends and neighbours, learn much from the feelings that Louise expresses – we should never deny the existence of a stillborn child. This mother is now receiving bereavement counselling and finding it useful. GPs will help to put their patients in touch with such counsellors.

Louise
Fifteen weeks ago I gave birth to twin boys. Sadly, one of my
sons, Ryan, was stillborn. This devastating news came after
eleven years of infertility and various forms of treatment.

When we finally got IVF treatment, our first attempt was
successful. Three embryos were implanted and two began to
develop. I was quite nervous, but also thrilled to be pregnant.
I felt really special, and told anyone who would listen that I was
expecting twins. My family were delighted, as were my friends.
I was given cribs and clothes, and all sorts of equipment; I had
to buy very little. I joined the local twins club and met other
mothers of twins who were very encouraging and supportive.
We bought an old twin pram and spent weeks cleaning it up.

At just over 36 weeks, I went into labour. I was in hospital
for the third time in my pregnancy. I went to the toilet, and as
I wiped myself I noticed a dark green discharge. I called a
midwife. They monitored the babies' heartbeats, and one of
them had gone down to 20 beats a minute. I had an emergency
Caesarean, but it was too late; Ryan never breathed.

The moments leading up to the operation were the most
frightening of my whole life. I was being shaved, having needles
put into me, a mask pushed on to my face all at the same time.
There was no one in the theatre I knew. I was sick, and someone
put their hand across my throat to stop it. I was crying and
praying for them to save my babies, but trying not to in case I
made things worse. When I came round, my husband Colin told
me that one of the babies was dead. I just remember screaming
over and over again, 'No, No, No.'

That day passed in a whirl. The baby who died, Ryan, was in
the room with us all day, but I can't remember. I held him, but
I can't remember. I have a photo that a midwife took of him,
but I wished she had taken one of me holding him.

Kyle was in Special Care. They brought him down to see me,
and I remember thinking that he wasn't such a nice baby as
Ryan, probably because he was wriggling around with tubes
stuck down his nose and a drip in his arm, whereas Ryan had
been peaceful and calm. Now of course I feel guilty for thinking
that. I feel guilty for all the times in my pregnancy that I said
I wanted a boy and a girl, not two boys. I feel that somehow
Ryan didn't feel wanted. I also feel that somehow he didn't want
me as a mother, or that I wouldn't have been able to cope with
two babies, so I was only allowed one.

When we went to Ryan's funeral, again I was in a state of shock. As we were walking up towards this tiny white coffin, I said to my husband, 'We shouldn't be here, we shouldn't be having to go to our baby's funeral.' It was how I felt when we were leaving the hospital. Colin was taking a photo of us with the midwife. I was crying and saying, 'I should be bringing two babies home.'

People say the most ridiculous things to us: 'At least you have one baby,' and 'You're only upset because of your hormones.' But the worst thing that people can do is pretend that it hasn't happened. Some people haven't even acknowledged the fact that Ryan existed. They have sent letters saying, 'Congratulations on the birth of your son.' I HAD TWO SONS. That's what I feel like shouting at them.

I am having bereavement counselling each week, which I think helps. The rage I feel at times is overwhelming. So is the sadness. I can be feeling absolutely fine, then something will trigger a memory and I'm off. I also feel that I shouldn't be talking about it to my friends and family. I feel like they will get fed up with hearing it. Also, my husband doesn't seem to feel as bad as I do. After the first couple of days he was able to accept it and get on with life. I am getting on with life, I have no choice as I have a young baby to look after, but it is not easy. To start with, I had long bouts of crying, my milk supply would diminish, which of course led to more problems. I felt that if I cried for Ryan, I could not feed Kyle, which made me feel guilty.

When I was about 33 or 34 weeks' pregnant, I went to my doctor with a watery discharge. He didn't examine me but said, 'It sounds like thrush.' It turned out that my waters had broken. Because of this, an infection got in and Ryan died of pneumonia.

In the following report Deborah puts across her beliefs very strongly, and she certainly has a point. Her son was stillborn at 24 weeks gestation which, at the time, was classified both medically and legally as a miscarriage. With changes to the abortion law and the increased survival chances of some foetuses (aided by intensive special care), the law was altered on 1 October 1992, reducing the age of 'viability' from 28 weeks to 24 weeks. This makes it difficult to perform straight comparisons between stillbirth rates before and after that time. In England and Wales, the legal definition of a stillbirth is 'a baby born dead after 24 completed weeks gestation or more'. In Scotland, the definition is 'a child which had issued forth from its mother after the twenty fourth week of pregnancy and which did not breathe or show any other sign of life'. The cut-off point in Northern Ireland is also 24 weeks. SANDS has provided the figures for stillbirths in 1993 given in Table 2. Figures for 1994 are provisional, but it seems likely that there was a slight decrease in England and Wales and in Scotland, and a slight increase in Northern Ireland, leading to an overall rate of 5.8.

Table 2   Stillbirths in the UK, 1993 (by area)

	England & Wales	Scotland	Northern Ireland	UK total
No. of stillbirths	3,855	409	130	4,394
Stillbirths per 1,000 births	5.7	6.4	5.2	5.7

At whatever point in a pregnancy that a baby dies, what is most important is that the medical staff involved are sensitive to the needs of the parents, using thoughtful terminology. Clearly, Deborah would have taken comfort from being able to christen and bury her child.

Deborah
When I was 20 weeks pregnant with my second child, I started to bleed and was sent by my GP to hospital. I was admitted for bed rest for about ten days.

A few weeks later I felt a slight dampness down below. I was visiting my GP for my antenatal that afternoon so thought nothing of this. At my appointment, the doctor seemed unconcerned but said he would send one of the local midwives around to my house to test if it was actually amniotic fluid leaking. No midwife turned up that evening.

At around 5am I was woken by severe pains. The doctor was called and asked a few questions, then left after giving me two very large tablets for wind and instructions to call when the surgery opened if the pain was no better. The pain was no better by then, so my husband called the surgery and said I was still in pain. Later that morning the doctor arrived, followed by the midwife who was coming to test for amniotic fluid leakage. I was sent immediately to hospital by ambulance. There I was told that I was in labour and that nothing could be done to stop it as my waters were broken.

I was given drugs, which I did not really want, but was told that as the foetus was already dead there seemed no point in having the pain. Later that day my son was born at 24 weeks, and this is the point from which I think the law and hospital procedure needed to be changed. We were asked if we wished to see the baby. We said yes and he was wheeled to us on a metal trolley wrapped up in a blanket, and put at the side of my bed. He lay there on that trolley; he was perfect in every way; he was a BABY! But because a foetus was not called a baby until 28 weeks gestation, then as far as they were concerned he was a miscarriage. We touched him and kissed him and then he was taken away.

The next morning I was visited by one of the nurses who asked if I had a photograph of my son, and when I said no went to ask about this. She came back saying that it was too late to take one, and that because we had seen him at the time and didn't ask for one, they didn't bother. For goodness sake! We had just lost a baby and we were supposed to ask if anyone had a camera handy. How ridiculous.

Later that day I was put on a side ward, which really finished me off. At least while in the ward I had other things on my mind, one being my friend who was brought in having a miscarriage at twelve weeks. I stood it for a few hours and asked to be discharged.

With the help of those around me, especially my friend who had the miscarriage, I managed to cope with my loss. Some time later, my sister lost her child at 38 weeks. This event brought everything back to me. The one main thing that stood out was that her son was christened and given a proper burial. Why could not these things be done for my baby? Babies were frequently surviving at 24 weeks and at this age they are no less a human being than they are at full term. Hospitals should be made more aware of parents' needs. We had no idea what the procedure was – for all we know, we may have been able to have our son christened and to have him taken away for a private burial. Your mind simply is not working properly, especially if, as I was, you have been given drugs to numb your senses. By the day after his birth, it sounds as though our son's body had already been disposed of, so even if we had thought of it then, it would have been too late.

After this I had three years of tests because I was having trouble conceiving and was sick to the back teeth of hearing, 'Oh yes, you had a miscarriage' – well, no, as far as I am concerned I had a stillborn baby. We did have another son four years later; he was born six weeks early and weighed just 4.5 lb (2.05kg). I still mourn every year on the day I lost our son, but this is not shared by anyone else because as far as the world is concerned, he never was a baby.

Deborah has perhaps found some retrospective comfort from the fact that the law has since changed and her loss would now be recognised as a stillbirth.

Janet discusses an issue which many mothers feel, but few are willing to talk about. She describes her initial emotions on hearing of the death of her baby as 'relief that I wouldn't have to look after the baby, because like most first-time mothers, I had worried how I would cope'. This initial, artificial relief was quickly followed by guilt at her 'betrayal of my baby', and this guilt is an inevitable feature of bereavement. Louise, writing earlier, also spoke of her guilt at having wished her twins were a boy and a girl rather than two boys, and for worrying that she wouldn't be able to cope with twins. The eventual stillbirth of one of her twin boys was, she felt, a result of her thoughts. Rationality tells us that such consequences cannot be attributed to earlier thoughts, but all rational thought can disappear under the shock of loss.

Janet has clearly coped well with her bereavement and gives thanks to her mother for listening patiently to her outpourings. Many of our writers have mentioned their need to talk at length of their loss, and those who have someone free to listen have, without exception, benefited from it.

Janet
I became pregnant for the first time and had a trouble-free 40 weeks; I was admitted to hospital at full term as my blood pressure was slightly raised and I had not put on any weight in the last three months. Labour was induced by a pessary and I was expected to go into labour the following day.

However, I quickly experienced severe pains and bleeding and after several hours was sent to the delivery suite. There were numerous staff in attendance and a foetal monitor showed my baby was in distress. By this time my husband, Peter, had been called from home. I was eventually told I would have a Caesarean.

When I was woken, the midwife told me that I had had a little girl, but that she had died during the operation because the placenta had separated from the uterus and caused a large clot to form. Therefore the baby had been deprived of oxygen. My immediate feeling was relief that I wouldn't have to look after the baby because, like most first-time mothers, I had worried how I would cope. Afterwards, I hated myself for that feeling – it seemed a betrayal of my baby.

Gradually, as the anaesthetic wore off, I felt the first waves of shock and grief. The consultant came and explained what had happened and the chaplain visited and said some prayers with us. Then the midwife and Peter washed and dressed Laura Fiona, and I held her and we had some photos taken.

All too soon, she was taken away to the mortuary and I never saw her again – now one of my greatest regrets. I had particularly wanted a girl but of course not a dead one. After all, babies don't die – not in hospital anyway. Laura was 5lb 12oz, perfect but dead.

I felt I had wasted all my good healthcare and had fallen at the last hurdle. Peter was able to stay in my room and we cried rivers.

The chaplain was wonderful and summed it all up – 'You've had an operation, got no baby and have the milk to feed her.' It wasn't surprising I felt desperately sad.

I was full of doubts and recriminations. I felt it must have been someone's fault and particularly hated the registrar for not doing an earlier Caesarean. It didn't change anything, though – Laura was still dead. The days passed quickly, with funeral arrangements to be made and friends and relatives to be informed.

I remember my mother-in-law visiting me at the hospital and me saying sorry to her. I also had a group of visitors one afternoon, and they all started chatting to each other and I got very irritated and wanted to cry out, 'Hey, our baby's died here, you know!'

We were assigned a social worker but he only visited a few times. I desperately needed to go over and over it again and again. I was later put into contact with another mum whose first baby died in almost identical circumstances and she was a terrific support and comfort.

I felt a lot of hurt over trivial things, like not having any baby cards or gifts. I suppose I had to focus my anger on something. In fact, I felt like a leper. I would peer into the other wards at the mums who were real mums as they had live babies.

After six days I was discharged, although I had a womb infection. Laura's pram stood empty except for a fluffy white rabbit we had bought on holiday while I was pregnant.

The tiny size of Laura's coffin came as a shock – like a large white shoebox. She was buried with two pink rosebuds, one from myself and one from Peter. There was a feeling of unreality about the birth and funeral and associated events – more like it was happening to someone else. No one should have to bury their baby – it's just not the natural sequence of life events.

I was glad of the physical discomfort of the Caesarean – it somehow kept me associated with my baby. I missed being pregnant and, in a way, found pregnant women more upsetting than babies – after all, I'd only really known the pregnancy.

After Peter returned to work there was a terrible void; although he was desperately upset too, he had his career to fill his days. I felt cheated and hurt – my future had been snatched away. Everyone knew what had happened but didn't want to say anything about it. The joy was taken out of everything.

I scoured the library and bookshelves for information and explanations. My mum was my greatest comfort – she had been dreadfully upset too and let me ramble on and on about it.

I knew everyone was willing us to try again for another baby, but my feelings were very complex. Not only did I have my original anxieties about parenthood but by now I was 35 and worried about amniocentesis, miscarriage, a further stillbirth. Basically, would it all go wrong a second time?

It is perhaps helpful to hear of my second pregnancy and childbirth. My pregnancy was confirmed by the first anniversary of Laura's death. It was a relief to know the decision was made, and there was no turning back. My mum was so pleased – she'd feared Laura's death would put me off ever trying again.

I had an almost identical pregnancy second time around, except I had a show at 26 weeks and had to have a week's hospital bed rest. This was a chance to reacquaint myself with the hospital and staff and try to banish some ghosts.

Throughout the pregnancy, I didn't dare hope for too much. Someone had told me it would be like walking on glass for nine months and they were right.

I was booked in for an elective epidural Caesarean at 38 weeks, but this baby had had enough of my anxiety by 37 weeks and I awoke in the night to find I was haemorrhaging.

Throughout the whole trip to the hospital, I was thinking that the placenta had detached again and it was going to be a repeat of the first time. When the monitor showed the baby's heartbeat, I was very happy but still very anxious. The registrar was a charming lady and we decided upon a general anaesthetic for an immediate Caesarean to save waiting for an epidural to work.

I was dreaming when the midwife woke me to say that I had had a little girl. I asked if she was alright and she was – 6 lb 4oz (2.84kg), perfect and alive. I had really wanted a girl and didn't know how I would have felt if it was a boy.

There was much joy at the birth of Caroline Rosie but much sadness too. I was in the same building where it had all gone wrong. It was only when Caroline was born and now as she is growing up that I really know what my loss was all about, even though I was desperately sad when my first baby died.

Every day I was afraid Caroline might be taken from us too. Sometimes, when she is asleep, I think she looks like her sister. It's hard not knowing what my baby would have grown up to be; to me she'll always be a baby. It is still difficult for me to accept friends having straightforward births. I know I have not fully come to terms with my baby's death, but I am learning to live with it.

Our next extract comes from Debbie, who tells the tale of her daughter Hayley, who died very shortly after her birth, and how she and her husband were asked if they would like to see Hayley after she died. They refused, but were persuaded by kind and sensitive staff that they would probably regret it later if they did not see her. Debbie was shown a photograph, which made her realise immediately that she must spend time saying goodbye to her daughter. It seems to be a recurring theme that parents of stillborn children are afraid of what they might see – the fear of deformity is one that haunts most of us, and yet a photograph, introducing the baby to his or her parents, can often begin to help

form a bond between parents and child, which helps enormously
in the long run.

Debbie
My first miscarriage was at 22 weeks, the second at 24 weeks.
My third loss was in August 1992. I had a little girl at 29 weeks
and we called her Hayley. She was perfect in every way, and very
tiny. She lived for just one hour. The medical services did
everything they could for her, but she was too weak to pull
through. When Hayley died, the midwife asked my husband and
me if we would like to see her. We didn't – I think we were very
confused and unwilling to accept what had happened. The
midwife told us that we would regret it if we did not see her now,
and she brought in a picture of Hayley. As soon as I saw the
picture I knew that I had to be with her. They brought her in
and I held her for a while. I am so glad now that I did, because
I certainly would have regretted doing otherwise and I will
always have a picture of her in my mind. The staff also took a
few more pictures of her, one where I was holding her, and I
find these photographs very comforting.

As I had had an emergency Caesarean which knocked me for
six, I felt at the time that I hated everyone, except my family.
For three days in hospital I saw Hayley often, so that I would
be able to remember every little detail of her. My husband
only saw her once – that was all he could handle. I know it
sounds silly, but I felt that she would sense it if I didn't go and
see her. All my family went to see her too, and that helps
because they know what Hayley looked like and we can all talk
about her – after all, she did exist.

I stayed in hospital for five days. I could have gone home
earlier but for some reason I did not want to go. In hospital I
felt secure, and the staff let my husband stay with me, which
was a great help. When I finally came out of hospital I felt I
should have been walking out with our baby, and that is when
I started to get very depressed. I was afraid to go anywhere just
in case people stopped me and asked whether I had a boy or a
girl, or else people might say, 'Never mind, better luck next time.'
In actual fact I found that people ignored me, which was just
as bad.

The next thing we had to cope with was the funeral. We had
Hayley buried, so every week we go to the cemetery, which helps
a lot. The first week when we went to the graveside, I felt

angry because I felt somehow that I should be visiting Hayley in Special Care, not in a cemetery.

I found myself unable to go out alone; someone had to be with me. When my husband went back to work, my mother would come over every morning at 7.30 and sit with me until the afternoon, when my sister arrived, and she would stay until my husband came home. I just could not be left alone. It helped enormously just having them there, even if we only sat quietly. It's so hard to explain how I felt. Sometimes I wanted to be with Hayley and other times I kept thinking life has to go on – as a lot of people told me.

I found that another thing that helped me through was the work of a colleague (Chris Jones) who organised a sponsored biathlon, with the winner getting the Hayley Reynolds Memorial Trophy. The race will be repeated each year and last year we raised £620 for the Scoo-B-Doo (Special Care Baby Unit Charity). It is nice to know that the money is going to help other special babies. Chris is also running the London Marathon and will get sponsors for Scoo-B-Doo.

My cousin's baby was due two days after Hayley and she had a little girl, and I find this very difficult to cope with. When she was pregnant she would come and visit me, but I found it hard to speak to her, in case I said anything that would worry her. Also, it reminded me that I should still be pregnant. Equally, when I went out and saw other mothers with babies, I would think it should be me. When my cousin gave birth I sent her a card, unable to visit. I know that she was very upset, and finally I plucked up the courage to go and see her. I was OK until the baby cried, and then I started to cry too, thinking that my baby never had the chance to do that.

I lost my fourth baby at twelve weeks, and for some reason I accepted this better. I started to bleed and immediately knew that something was wrong. I went to the hospital and a scan showed that I was losing my baby yet again. When they told me I cried. It was probably too soon after losing Hayley – I became pregnant in two months – but I felt I just had to have a baby. I have decided now to wait a while before I try again – I don't think I was ready, mentally or physically. I am confident that one day I will have children, because I can't give up.

It is the support of my family that has kept me sane through these times, and I know how lucky I am to have them. Also, I begin to realise that you are not alone – we went to a memorial service at the hospital for parents of lost babies and the church was packed. Still, I feel very empty.

Incidentally, there is a footnote to Debbie's account. She wrote to us at the time of going to press to let us know that she now has a lovely little girl, Pippa, born in 1994.

Ruth mentions an aspect of stillbirth that terrifies many of us – after discovering that the baby she was carrying had died in the womb, she experienced 'a feeling of revulsion' at the thought of the dead child inside her. And yet Ruth bravely underwent labour to deliver her baby, finding strength she did not know she possessed, feeling the need to experience the final contact with her baby. She speaks with praise of the professionals who attended her, although she regrets the fact that she did not have a chance to spend time touching her dead daughter.

Ruth
My daughter Claire's birth was for me a healing process after the cot death of my son, Stewart, and when she was two and a half years old I returned to work, feeling that at last my life had taken on a semblance of normality. But soon I discovered that I was pregnant once more. Initially I was not too happy, but eventually I accepted this.

The last thing I expected was any sort of complication with this pregnancy, and therefore I was not aware of every kick and turn that the developing foetus made. When I eventually realised that the movements had in fact slowed down considerably, it may have been too late for Maria's life to be saved. When, at last, I was told that our daughter had died in the womb, my husband was at work, totally oblivious to the trauma that was unfolding. I really could not believe that a second baby of ours had ceased to live in such a sudden and shocking way. I felt I was being meted out for some kind of divine punishment – perhaps I had not wanted this baby enough?

A feeling of revulsion soon swamped every fibre of my body as I realised I was now a walking coffin and may even be carrying some terrible monster who was, at that very moment, decomposing inside me.

Paradoxically, I needed to experience the forthcoming labour totally and absolutely, as I realised this would be the final contact I would have with our baby. Thankfully, because of the tender, loving care that we received from all the professionals that we encountered, it was a positive and profound experience.

My only regret is that I never touched Maria; fear of the unknown prevented me from doing so. If only I had been given time to confront the feelings that stopped me from touching my daughter, but she was whisked away for a post-mortem which revealed no apparent cause of death – once again we were left with questions that would never be answered. This second loss seemed, in some ways, harder to bear than the first one.

A stillbirth is such a lonely grief. When Stewart had died, I could share his life with so many people, but I was the only one that had known our daughter – not even my husband had felt her growing as I had. I yearned to hold and feed her as I had imagined – I would never know the colour of her eyes or give her comfort when she needed it. The pain and agony of this second loss plunged me into such depths of grief that there were times when I believed I would never have the strength to climb out again.

When I became pregnant once more, I was hopeful that all would be well but at 14 weeks I lost the baby. If this had been our first miscarriage, I would have experienced all the usual symptoms of bereavement, but all I felt was a sense of disappointment – this loss could not and would not touch me.

There was, thankfully, a happy ending. For a year after the miscarriage, I attempted to become pregnant; my whole being focused on this one goal.

Finally, I found that I was expecting a baby. As I was regarded as a 'high-risk' pregnancy, I was closely monitored throughout the next eight months, a time that was filled with a whole gamut of emotions ranging from absolute panic to a tranquil realisation that all would be well this time.

Isabel was born by Caesarean section. She had not been developing as well as she should have been and my consultant felt that to leave her would have been too risky.

I was conscious for Isabel's arrival, for I needed to see and acknowledge that here, at last, was the baby that I had yearned for. There were emotional problems after Isabel's birth – initially, a difficulty in separating Isabel and Maria: they were, for me, one baby, and if I tried to entangle their identities I was consumed with a sense of betrayal.

Susan writes with heartwarming sincerity of the battle she and her son, Matthew, fought for life. Her much-wanted child lived for five days and she treasures the memory.

Susan

What a surprise I had when I found out that I was pregnant for the fifth time at the ripe old age of 42. I was worried about the reactions of my other children, aged 21, 19, 15 and a special little boy aged 9 who has mild cerebral palsy. But they were over the moon about it.

We were anxious because I had had a difficult fourth pregnancy, needing to stay in hospital for over eight months. My GP was worried and offered me a termination, but I longed to have this baby. The pregnancy was difficult, needing several hospital admissions, but the consultant and the hospital were great. I was shown how to give myself injections twice a day of a drug called heparin. This was to keep my blood thin, as I had developed a blood clot in my leg.

When I was 16 weeks pregnant I had an alphafetoprotein test and I was told I would need an amniocentesis. I had to wait an anxious three long weeks for the result but, thank goodness, the result came back as normal.

When I reached 27 weeks I became quite poorly. I was transferred from the maternity hospital to the coronary care unit. I was very short of breath and the doctors said I had developed a blood clot in my lungs. They had to give me drugs and yet more heparin in a drip.

Unfortunately, the drugs made me bleed inside my stomach. For three days I was in a lot of pain. The doctors had to operate to save my life and I was rushed back to the maternity hospital. There were 4 litres of blood in my stomach and Matthew was in breech position and in distress. They had to take him out of the womb at 29 weeks. He was so small and helpless. They rushed him to Special Care. They all loved him down on the unit. His Special Nurse cared for him so much. Because I was in intensive care, fighting for my life, I was not able to see him straight away. We knew there was not much hope and the doctors warned me to expect the worst, but we hung on to the slightest improvement only to be put down the next day or even the next hour. I longed to tell him how much we all loved him, to hold him and cuddle him.

When they were able to take me down to see him, they had to arrange the Special Care room so they could get my bed in with all the equipment and monitors attached to me. At first I could not look at him. I did not want to love him; he was so frail and helpless. We had him christened and the nurses dressed him up in a lovely white gown. We were all there. My nine-year-old son held his little hand inside the incubator.

Things went well for a couple of days, but then he developed infection after infection. The drugs I had taken in pregnancy had made him bleed inside too. His dad never left his side. He talked to him and stroked his tiny body, willing him to live. But two days later he had a bleed into his brain and the doctors said there was no hope. They asked us to turn the ventilator off.

We had Matthew for five days. Everybody loved him. He died in his big brother's arms, with us all around him. I just wish I had been well enough to hold him and dress him and tell him how much we all wanted him.

The doctors let me out of hospital to attend his funeral. His tiny teak coffin made me cry. The church was packed with all our friends and family, and his little grave is always covered with flowers that people have kindly put there. We did not have him for very long, but I truly loved that baby, more than I can ever say. On my bad days, I still blame myself for Matthew's early death, but I have found talking to other mothers at a SANDS meeting helpful.

The hospital gave me lots of photos of Matthew and I also found this helpful as I had little time with my son. I wish I could have got to know him better. I know that Matthew will be my last baby. Deep down, I long for another pregnancy but my age is against it. I just wish I did not have to end my childbearing years like this; and yes, I do know I am very lucky to have four children already and I thank God every day for them.

Somehow, the next account needs no introduction, no explanation. We feel it sums up perfectly the emotions and experiences of a stillbirth, and we will not spoil it with analysis, but use this remarkable piece of writing to end this chapter.

Tricia

I had a relatively uneventful pregnancy, followed by an emergency Caesarean section by epidural anaesthetic. It followed exactly the same pattern as that of my previous delivery: in fact my son (now three years old) was in rather a worse condition than our daughter by the end of labour – he survived and scored a healthy 9 on the Apgar scale [the Apgar ratings are explained in the Glossary]. I could feel our daughter's movements right up to the theatre doors. A few minutes later she was delivered and I heard no cries. Another paediatrician was summoned, then the senior registrar. All the while, the surgeon stitching my tummy was reassuring – the more acute the case, the faster our daughter was bound to recover. I overheard such phrases as 'still flat', 'blood Ph7.8', 'I tried intubating twice'. My husband's face told the whole story, and when the senior registrar approached I knew what she was going to say.

I was absolutely confounded: it couldn't, simply didn't, happen these days. The perinatal death rate for the hospital was 40 in 6,000 births per annum. She was the wished-for daughter – there must have been some mistake. She couldn't be dead. Not *our* baby. The theatre staff wept with us.

I was quickly wheeled into the recovery room. Our daughter was placed in a crib beside us. She was perfect, simply sleeping in repose. My husband and I took it in turns to hold her. Two midwives were assigned to stay with us and the Anglican chaplain arrived quickly to bless her and name her. The baby was washed, dressed and placed in a Moses basket. The staff admired her, pointing out her features, shape, the colour of her hair, how much she resembled us. We had photographs taken, and keep other precious mementoes.

Our sense of loss was immediate: we regretted the things that she would never do, the part we had allotted her in our lives that would never be played out, milestones she would never reach, the love and support we would never be able to give her.

I held her close, wanting to keep her warm. We thought we saw a flicker of an eyelid, the rise and fall of her chest. My mother later cuddled her as naturally as if she had been alive. This experience of being with her after her death for five or more hours was undoubtedly the most significant part of the whole tragedy: afterwards, we started beginning to integrate her into our lives. It meant that I was able to accept the reality of her being and her death, that she had really existed as well as the terrible fact of her lost potential. The hospital staff showed so much kindness and compassion at every stage, but especially at this time.

It was suggested that I be moved to an antenatal ward, but I requested an ordinary maternity ward. I needed to be with mothers and their babies – I could at least recall the joy and excitement of having my first baby and a reminder of my son waiting at home.

My husband and I found ourselves surrounded by love and genuine help: first and foremost from our families. My in-laws came to stay until two days after my discharge and cared for my husband and son. Friends and neighbours rallied around with messages of support, flowers, cakes and letters. Colleagues called after seeing the birth announcement. What surprised us was the commonality of experience – how many friends and acquaintances had suffered the same devastation and yet never spoke of it.

Most of all, our faith has come to our aid. The chaplain asked, 'Do you blame God?' It seems illogical for God to destroy potential professors of His faith – why should a shepherd sacrifice his lambs? He showed His concern for the human condition by sending His son to die on the cross. Until this century, perinatal death was a common fact of everyday life and the faith survived unquestioned through the generations.

The vicar at our old home gladly complied with our wish to have our daughter buried at the church at which we were married and where our son was baptised. Mercifully, the law has changed in this respect over the past three years and we were able to give her a permanent and consecrated resting place. I felt an enormous sense of calm and comfort when helping arrange her funeral service.

We trusted our instincts too. One counsellor suggested it might be a good idea for our three-year-old to see our daughter two days after her death: the reasoning seemed to be that he might not otherwise understand our grief, and could feel guilty. He had displayed uncharacteristically destructive behaviour at home while I was away, but it later proved to be maternal deprivation that was his main concern, rather than the death of an unknown sibling. I can appreciate that an older child may have the power to understand loss, but I would caution other people in our position to be wary of psycho-babble. In the event, he is just beginning to ask relevant questions, which we try to answer as they arise. A child's psyche is enormously complex (and largely uncharted), but need not be reinterpreted to suit particular theories at every turn.

The initial post-mortem report showed a pulmonary problem, but many questions remain unanswered. Is it worse to know that one has carried an abnormal baby or a healthy child who died inexplicably during labour? Was the labour mismanaged, and would earlier intervention have saved our daughter? No amount of rationale or compensation, no dismissals or cautions could possibly replace her.

We have tried to do the things in death for her we could not do in life: giving her the names we'd chosen, placing her toys with her, burying her in a place sacred to us – and other details which will unfold over the next months. And the mother–child relationship still holds, even when mother and child are separated: the longing to hold her, the irrational concern that she may be cold, lonely or hungry. Through this period of shock and numbness there is simply a void, a great 'why?': no rhyme or reason why a beloved baby should be taken from us. We thought ourselves blessed, and found that we were bereft.

3 Medical problems which may be a factor

It is hard to imagine the shock and pain caused by the discovery late in a pregnancy, or on the birth of a child, that one's baby has a life-threatening illness. Labour is a traumatic event even when it goes well, and for the new parents the worry caused by news of a baby's health problem must shake them to the core. It is not our place to judge whether it is worse to experience the birth of a live but terminally ill baby, or to have a baby stillborn. The former inevitably allows the parents briefly to welcome their child, but equally may offer them a cruel hope which is all too soon snatched away.

It is doubtful that there is ever much comfort in knowing the cause of a baby's death. As one contributor writes, 'Is it worse to know that one has carried an abnormal baby or a healthy child who died inexplicably during labour?' Perhaps the only benefit to be gained by parents from the knowledge of the cause of their baby's death is where it offers reassurance that the same thing is unlikely to happen again.

The potential causes of the death of a baby around the time of its birth are numerous. If one were to ask 100 pregnant women what health concerns they have for their baby, there would probably be 100 different answers. We are not attempting here to be in any way a medical textbook. We are not qualified to proffer medical advice, nor would we want to. Our aim, rather, is to offer an opportunity to those people who have suffered loss to share their experience with others. Readers will note just how often contributors write that at the time of their suffering they felt utterly alone, convinced that no one else had ever before felt the emotions they were experiencing.

This chapter identifies some causes of stillbirth and neonatal death. Each contributing parent tells us a little about the particular illness that struck their child, and we have expanded this information with details available from the various support organisations. In chapter 8 we provide details of relevant groups, so that any readers with specific anxieties can contact those people who have the knowledge to provide practical help.

Pre-eclampsia

Pre-eclampsia is a condition specific to pregnancy, the cause of which is still unknown. It is indicated when two of the following three symptoms are present:

- raised blood pressure;
- swelling of the feet, ankles and hands;
- protein in the urine.

This condition very seldom occurs before the twentieth week of pregnancy and is nearly always associated with extra weight gain. The essential change is a rise in blood pressure. The normal pressure in a healthy 25-year-old woman is around 120/70mm and does not alter greatly in normal pregnancy. The second, lower (diastolic) figure changes if there is a fundamental alteration in the body, and in cases of pre-eclampsia rises to about 90.

As a result of the raised blood pressure, protein is shed from the kidneys and can be detected in the urine. Routine urine tests are performed at every antenatal visit partly to detect the presence of protein. Pre-eclampsia is one of many reasons why protein is found in the urine during pregnancy.

Pre-eclampsia develops slowly and insidiously, but can usually be diagnosed by stringent antenatal care and can then be treated. If, for whatever reason, this does not happen, pre-eclampsia can become eclampsia, which is extremely dangerous to both mother and child.

The real danger of pre-eclampsia is to the unborn child. It has been estimated that in the United Kingdom approximately 7 per cent of women having their first babies and 3 per cent of those having subsequent babies suffer from pre-eclampsia – sometimes with disastrous results to their babies. The danger to the baby varies directly with the increase in the mother's diastolic blood pressure. Premature labour, either spontaneous or induced, results in a high proportion of small babies so that almost 10 per cent of these babies fail to survive.

Sandra offers the following report. Her son, Lloyd, was born prematurely and seriously ill after Sandra developed pre-eclampsia. It is clear from her own words that she and her husband felt that her pregnancy and subsequent care should have been handled very differently. Indeed, the birth of their second son was dealt with, in a different hospital, much more to Sandra's liking. It is worth noting that because it was known that this mother was prone to high blood pressure, her second pregnancy was monitored and she was treated accordingly to produce a small, but healthy, child. It is also of interest that Sandra and her husband visited a geneticist after losing their first son – such a course should have worked to reassure them and it is unfortunate that the visit was mismanaged, sidetracked by an analysis of Lloyd's death, while the parents just wanted to move forwards.

Lloyd's death is not medically classified as neonatal, for he was clearly a fighter and managed to live for four months. However, many similar cases do result in babies dying much sooner after birth.

Sandra

I became pregnant in June and was registered at the doctor's as having normal blood pressure. However, by the end of October it had started to rise and the doctor was seeing me fortnightly. No one told me anything about high blood pressure and the problems which go with it.

I saw a consultant and he admitted me straight away into hospital. He, and his nurse, wouldn't tell me what the BP was at the time (140/105), and it wasn't until I left in mid-January that I found out.

I was putting on weight during all this time, but I had no big lump, just a large tummy. I had a routine scan at 16 weeks and a scan a week after I was admitted to hospital. I was supposedly 29 weeks pregnant, but the baby was showing as 25 weeks and weighing 1lb 8oz-1lb 10oz (0.68-0.73kg).

The week beginning 8 January, a house doctor told me that a Caesarean section would be done on the Friday. He told me that the baby would be small, but his lungs would be quite good as he had been fighting for his life. I was also advised to go and see round the Special Care Baby Unit (SCBU). Another scan showed the baby had grown slightly and was now approximately

1lb 12oz–2lb (0.8–0.9kg).The radiographer then informed my
husband David and myself that our baby had stopped growing
and no further explanation was given.

On the Tuesday night my husband left me at about 9 o'clock
and I went to bed, but later had the most awful sharp stabbing
pains in my back. In the morning I still didn't feel well and by
4 o'clock that afternoon they decided to do an emergency
Caesarean section. I later found out that this was to save me and
not the baby. The stabbing pains in my back had been my
kidneys starting to give up.

By the time my husband arrived, I was gowned and being
wheeled down to theatre. No one bothered to tell him anything,
and he was left outside not knowing what was going on, until
the consultant came out and said, 'It's a girl, but don't hold your
hopes up,' and just walked off.

The SCBU nurses soon came out with a scrap of a baby and
told David it was a boy and to follow them to SCBU. They were
all excellent; they did their tests, cleaned up Lloyd and then told
David what was going on. This was the first time someone had
spoken to us as human beings with feelings. They even arranged
for a polaroid to be given to me, as I was unable to see him for
18 hours. He weighed 1lb 6$\frac{1}{2}$oz (0.64kg) and was breathing on
his own. We later found out that when he was first born they
did have a problem to get him to breathe, and were just giving
up hope when he started.

On the Friday afternoon we had a meeting with Lloyd's
consultant. We were told that he only had a 5 per cent chance
of living and that they were unable to tell us for certain if he
was a boy or a girl, as his genitals were very enlarged and he had
no testicles.

The SCBU staff were extremely kind and helpful and
encouraged David and me to do as much of his day-to-day care
as we wanted. They even used to get Lloyd out of his incubator
and put him to my breasts, in order that he could get his
sucking reflexes working. He was fed through a naso-gastric tube
for the first few months, but I expressed my milk for four
months for him.

After three and a half weeks Lloyd was found to have a
hernia, and had to go to a larger hospital for an operation.

Lloyd then caught a cold at the end of February and he had
to be ventilated for one week. When he came off the ventilator

he had to be given oxygen and, other than the occasional breaks, he was on oxygen until he died.

Tests on Lloyd revealed that he was definitely a boy, but he did have a severe case of hypospadias (this is when a boy cannot urinate from the end of his penis).

The first real highlight was in April, taking Lloyd out for a walk. He was still on oxygen, but the staff rigged up an oxygen cylinder to his pram, and towards the end of the month he had actually given up oxygen. He then got another hernia, but in spite of this it was arranged that we could bring him home. I went and stayed in the hospital with him – they had a small mother's room just off SCBU. The hernia then got worse, and he was taken to yet another hospital and operated on. Again, a week later it was decided that I should go in and stay, with a view to bringing him home. But this time he ended up back on oxygen.

It was then decided to show me how to do physio on Lloyd, how to insert a naso-gastric tube and how to suck him out. This I learnt, and on 21 May I was again in the hospital getting ready for him to come home for the third time. Lloyd was now taking small amounts of solids and enjoying them, but he still had some problems with the bottles, and on 24 May at his night feed his breathing was very shallow and he was not his normal self. I took him back to SCBU and the doctors were called. He had aspirated his feed, which was duly sucked up. He was put back on oxygen and David and I went home, with Lloyd looking much better and breathing well.

26 May. This was the day that Lloyd should have come home. I phoned the hospital as soon as I awoke and was told that he was still on oxygen, but had had a good night. When I arrived at SCBU he was just staring into space and looked grey. I phoned David and told him to come to the hospital. Just after that call, Lloyd had a cardiac arrest. He was taken into the intensive care part of the SCBU and I was whisked to a waiting room just outside. Everyone was running in and out, even the midwives from the other floors, while I just had to sit there not knowing what was happening to my baby, feeling completely helpless. Yet again, no one told me what was going on. After a while I went to wait for David; as he drove into the hospital, I knew our very brave little boy had passed away.

David, who had been the strong one throughout the four and a half months, went to pieces, while I seemed suddenly to

gain his strength. We were able to hold Lloyd, alone, and then
we had him christened.

We were offered no counselling, but after a month I went to
the doctor's and he put us in touch with someone. This lady
has since set up a SANDS group. The hospital also has a chapel
and a book of remembrance was started that summer; we were
asked if we would like to make an entry, which we did and we
now have somewhere to visit.

Another source of comfort to me was the diary I kept from
1 January right the way through to June. I still look at it now
and then, and it is lovely to look back and remember the
happy times we shared with Lloyd.

It took me a long time to fall pregnant again, and I put this
down to all the pent-up loss. My next pregnancy was monitored
very, very carefully, but this is because I refused to go back to
the same hospital. When I was 38 weeks pregnant my blood
pressure shot up, and they gave me a pill to crack and dissolve
under my tongue. They also advised me to lie on my left side,
as this reduced pressure on the heart and therefore helped to
reduce the blood pressure. I now look back and wonder why
there is a simple procedure in one hospital, and none in the
other.

Our second child, Ashleigh, was also little. He weighed 4lb
9oz (2.07kg), so I take it that there is a problem with me
carrying a baby, but no one has ever suggested or told me
anything. We did see a geneticist after Lloyd died, but he only
seemed to want to give us a reason as to why Lloyd had died
(which he couldn't) and not as to why he was small and why
he had had so many problems, i.e. hypospadias, lung problems,
etc. He did a follow-up on Ashleigh, but still no reasons were
given as to why he was small. No tests were done on David,
Ashleigh or myself, if any are available.

I know that some of this sounds as if we are very bitter at
certain doctors who looked after me during my pregnancy, but
we are the sort of people who wanted to know everything that
was going on. It was the Catch-22 situation, the doctors thinking
too much information might cause problems and us wanting
to know but not knowing how to find out. In my case, my
consultant was of the *very* old school, i.e. he didn't want to
supply any information, or even talk to me, so as far as I was
concerned everything was continuing fine, even though the

baby appeared to be small, until the very end when it was obvious that things weren't right.

I think one of the ways forward would be that during their training doctors should be taught how to ask leading questions, which would help them find out how much information the patients wanted to know, what they could take in and how they would cope with the said information.

Growth retardation

In some pregnancies, the placenta grows but fails to mature properly and so produces less hormone than normal. This was historically referred to as placental insufficiency, but is now known medically as growth retardation. It has a direct effect on the entire pregnancy. The uterus remains consistently smaller than it should be, while the mother's weight gain is less than expected. The baby is smaller than average and there is only a small quantity of amniotic fluid present, offering less cushioning for the foetus.

This dysmature placenta can only provide a restricted supply of nutrition to the foetus, with the result that the baby develops normally but slowly. Eventually, inevitably, the placenta can no longer supply even the basic requirements and the baby becomes short of oxygen and may die in the womb.

It is also possible for a placenta to appear to function normally until the thirty-second to thirty-fourth week. After this there is rapid and unusual deterioration, due to factors that may or may not be recognised. The failure of the placenta to continue to work normally results in a slowing down of the baby's growth, until it ceases altogether. First, the baby's liver and spleen stop growing, then the baby accumulates less fat and finally the head stops growing. This last sign is associated with an increased risk of the baby dying in the womb, as well as increased perinatal mortality. The undernourished baby does not have sufficient glucose in its starved liver to withstand the stress of labour, and may become distressed. Occasionally this happens before labour, and an emergency Caesarean section may be required.

One of the main aims of the medical staff at antenatal classes is to recognise if a baby is not growing as it should. Modern scientific advances have made this easier.

The following case demonstrates a seemingly normal pregnancy that resulted in the birth of a dead baby. Growth retardation was assumed to be the cause – the baby did not have sufficient energy reserves to survive the trauma of birth.

This loss appears to have been handled with sensitivity and care – the staff produced a 'booklet', so providing something by which the grieving parents could remember their beloved daughter. The positive use of photographs can also be seen time and time again throughout the contributions.

Amanda
After a perfectly normal pregnancy, I awoke one night with the runs and I'd also had a show. I rang the hospital and was told that unless I was in any pain they were both quite normal. I wasn't suffering, so I went back to bed and awoke the following morning feeling fine. At 12.25 I had my first pain. I'd been told that first labours usually lasted a good 12–15 hours but by 1.40 pm my mother and I decided this was progressing too fast, with pains now every three minutes and lasting one minute. I got my husband home from work and at 2pm we set off on the half-hour journey to the hospital. By now the pains were every minute and lasting one minute. I wanted to push and we were only halfway there.

I managed to hang on and finally made it to the labour ward. Now I could push; no I couldn't. I was fully dilated but the head I could feel turned out to be a bottom; she was breech. I didn't have time to get undressed. The room was now a buzz of people: a doctor examining me, a midwife strapping me to a monitor (she couldn't find a heartbeat and three different people tried). I knew something was wrong, and they asked my husband to leave but he wouldn't. No one said anything. I lay there thinking they'd got it wrong, the baby must be laid wrongly. I began to panic. The doctor told me to push as the baby was here. They gave me gas and air; I think this was more to ease the panic than the pain. Looking back, I needed the pain because the rest of me was numb. Three pushes and the baby was born. She was rushed away; two minutes later she was back. She was beyond resuscitation; she'd been dead for a while. A doctor tried to fit a drip into my hand but I wanted my baby. I didn't even know if it was a boy or a girl. I held Andrew, who was sobbing uncontrollably, 'There is no baby, no baby.' I said, 'There is a baby. I want my baby.'

The questions began. The doctor was quite abrupt. When did I last feel her move? Had I had an infection? I felt her move yesterday, or had I imagined it? I didn't know. On Wednesday I was told she was engaged head down, and to go home and rest and not to worry as they don't move much at 39 weeks. I didn't want to answer their questions. I wanted my baby, and by now I was becoming desperate.

A nurse finally brought her over. She was beautiful, so perfect, yet so small at 4lb 14oz (2.22kg). I checked her over to make sure she had all her parts. The consultant came in and tried to explain that the placenta had stopped working and our baby wasn't being properly nourished and the oxygen supply was cut down, so when labour began she was already too tired to cope with the speed of it all, but tests would be done and a post-mortem carried out. We were moved into the SANDS room across the corridor from delivery. We were very lucky; it had only been finished a few weeks before.

I began to think. She must have been fed; I'd eaten all the right things, watched my diet, taken in lots of fresh air, didn't smoke or drink. This wasn't fair. I suddenly realised we didn't have a name. Andrew decided on Catherine because it meant 'pure' and she looked just that. Our parents arrived and were very upset. They couldn't understand why I wasn't, as I sat there in bed with my baby explaining what had happened. After our parents had gone, a nurse came in to take some photos of us together and of Catherine in the basket. She had also made a booklet, and did foot- and handprints and cut a lock of her hair. I cuddled my baby. Her skin was so smooth, her hair so dark. I talked to her and told her all the things I had planned to do. I still did not cry but I lay awake all night watching the clock. The ward was very busy that night and I heard every noise. Suddenly I heard a baby cry, and the awful truth hit me that it wasn't our baby. My baby didn't cry. She was dead. She was born silent; nothing would ever be the same again. I felt sick. I was suffocating, I couldn't breathe. Andrew held me and I cried and sobbed for hours. What had we done to deserve this? What did anybody do to deserve this?

I walked around with Catherine, nursing and rocking her, cuddling and crying on her. The nurse came in and said we could go home now. I didn't want to go home. Why couldn't I take my baby home? I felt so empty; normal people went home with babies. We left Catherine at the hospital to have the post-mortem and discussed the funeral arrangements on the way home. We decided to have a small service at the chapel of rest and have Catherine cremated so she could be with my grandma.

When I got home, I hated my body. I had no right to be fat: I had no baby, so no right to stretch marks, stitches and engorged bursting breasts. Our regular midwife was on holiday and the lady who came did her checks and went. The next week passed us by in a daze. When Friday came, we were relieved. We'd been in limbo all week waiting finally to say goodbye to our daughter. Catherine was in a tiny shoebox-sized coffin, in the clothes I had dressed her in, with a photo of Mummy and Daddy and a cuddly doll which had belonged to me as a child; I hoped my grandma would recognise this and take care of her. Andrew carried Catherine's crib into the crematorium and within minutes she was gone. The funeral director gave me a dark pink rose from our posy. A weight was lifted from us; Catherine was finally at peace, where no one could hurt her and she was already on her way to a better place. We have a plaque in the garden of remembrance and visit often with our pink roses.

My heart aches for my beautiful little girl and there is a void in our lives that can never be filled. I think about her every day, and love and miss her. It has taken me nearly three months to be able to talk about it.

Trisomy 18

Each human cell contains 22 pairs of chromosomes numbered 1 to 22, and one pair of sex chromosomes (XX in females, XY in males). The word 'trisomy' means three chromosomes of a kind, instead of the usual pair. The extra chromosome is already present in either the sperm or the egg at fertilisation, and is not caused during the pregnancy.

An extra chromosome 18 causes Trisomy 18, also called Edward's syndrome. The condition was formally known as E Trisomy. As with Down's syndrome (Trisomy 21) and Trisomy 13 (see below), the risk of giving birth to a baby with Trisomy 18 increases with maternal age. Except in rare cases that are inherited, chromosome defects are usually one-off events. Only rarely is there a previous history of such a birth. The degree of medical problems and disability involved can vary widely in children affected by partial or full trisomy, even if they have the same chromosome defect.

This is because the genetic material that is extra or missing is different in every case. Some babies with Trisomy 18 (and also Trisomy 13) suffer from major internal abnormalities and are stillborn.

Trisomy 18 affects one in 3,000 births and is three times more likely in girls than in boys. Extremely comprehensive booklets on Trisomy 18 (and Trisomy 13) and related disorders can be obtained from Soft UK – a support organisation whose address is given in chapter 8.

Sue
At 30 weeks, I went to my usual Wednesday morning antenatal clinic. Considering my dates, the doctor thought I didn't look pregnant enough. Privately, I had congratulated myself on this but I had a twinge of uneasiness when I was told to be at hospital in 30 minutes for a scan. Once there and after much hanging around, countless people scanning and prodding me, I was asked to return with my overnight things. Chris and I spent much of the next 36 hours sitting in a maternity ward. As I wasn't actually sick, they let me home at night. After endless scans, it was concluded that my baby, at 30 weeks gestation (and fortunately, I was convinced it was 30 weeks), had a head with a dimension of 27 weeks and an abdomen of 24 weeks. This suggested serious oxygen starvation, where development of the brain takes priority over the torso. I could see that sounded bad, but was still confident that I just had a small baby.

On Friday morning we were asked to go to a teaching hospital in London. It has the best foetal scanning skills in the region, and it was felt that we couldn't get better advice than there. Chris and I settled in for another big wait. I lay on various beds and was prodded, scanned and doppler scanned again. I was told the baby could be small for three reasons:

1. Normally small (and I was convinced it was this one).
2. Oxygen starvation due to an inefficient umbilical cord or placenta.
3. A chromosomal defect.

The person who did the doppler on me used the phrase 'seriously abnormal' to describe the baby's oxygen rates at about 3pm. At last I had to accept that this was more than a normally small baby. He showed that the baby's oxygen intake was impeded and that the carbon dioxide level was excessive. I then lay for at least another hour with a foetal heartbeat monitor pressed against me. At 5pm I was swept back to see the main mover in the unit, who mimed the unthinkable: I was going to have a Caesarean. Another bed, this time surrounded by about twelve people, a stab in the belly and off people rushed with umbilical blood samples for tests. Fears were confirmed. The tests indicated that the baby would die in the next few days due to oxygen starvation: only a week later, after chromosomal tests, would we know if there was a chromosomal problem. The baby couldn't wait to find out. We agreed to a Caesarean, suddenly finding that there was no real option. We were told the operation would be at 8pm that day, 'unless your baby becomes distressed, in which case it will be sooner'.

Chris supported me by being normal and enthusiastically dressed up in operation togs, including a ridiculous bonnet, and accompanied me to theatre. Very effortlessly for me, a baby was delivered. Immediately, about six gowned medics pored over this little scrap on her 'operating table'. Yes, a girl; we had hastily decided to call her Rachel Alexandra. From my prone position, I was given a glimpse of Rachel and then she disappeared to the Special Care Baby Unit (SCBU). Two hours later Chris was allowed to visit Rachel and came back with a polaroid of our daughter.

A mattress was installed for Chris in my bedroom and we slept uneasily. At midday it was decided that I could see my daughter. Getting into the wheelchair revealed to me how physically weak and sore I was, and by the time I reached SCBU I was emotionally wrecked. I sat in the chair with my knees in the way in front of Rachel's incubator, shattered by the journey and discovering post-Caesarean pain, looking at a 1lb 10oz (0.74kg) scrap, with ventilator, drips, splints, etc. comprising the greater part of my picture.

Although intellectually I accept the turn of events and understand that it had to happen to someone and it just happened to be us and Rachel, I have cried and cried and cried. After a week of optimism and my good recovery from the operation, we were told that in spite of looking reasonably normal Rachel did have a chromosomal problem. She had something called Trisomy 18 or Edward's syndrome, meaning that at the eighteenth chromosome pair she had three rather than two chromosomes, affecting her throughout her body. She would be physically and mentally retarded. Only 10 per cent of Edward's babies live to one year – i.e. 90 per cent die before. Because she was so young and so small, her lungs were poor and she relied on the ventilator: if she did not come off it in three months, she never would. She had a patent ductus, a shortcircuit just outside the heart, because of her prematurity, which worsened her lungs. Apparently, with Edward's syndrome there is no change in growth until after 20 weeks. I understand that all babies grow at the same rate up to that stage, but after the groundwork has been done most babies surge forward. It would only have been apparent that something was not quite right (but not necessarily wrong) in the last fortnight or so. The diagnosis of oxygen starvation was only confirmed after I was put on a doppler scan, where oxygen flow could be assessed. I also understand that as Rachel was an Edward's baby from the first splitting of the cells, the triple test could possibly have indicated her problem.

We decided we would visit Rachel daily. Our memories are of Wandsworth roadworks, the South Circular and the SCBU, and that evocative smell of disinfectant we used whenever we entered. We would spend maybe an hour just stroking the parts of Rachel we could reach, mostly her head, but sometimes a beautiful, soft, downy arm or leg. If we were there at the right time of day, we were encouraged to clean Rachel's lips and bottom and give her a new nappy. Many friends and relatives wanted to visit Rachel (which we liked) and at least 50 per cent of our visits were done with 'guests'; only by seeing Rachel in the flesh could one understand her smallness, her plight and also the personality which we gleaned from her inquisitive eyes, her expressive brow and the wrinkling of her bottom when we wiped it with wet cotton wool. I expressed milk four times a day and constantly hoped that 'next week' Rachel would be strong enough for it; in the meantime, she had a diet of glucose, minerals and lipids. After a month, Rachel had regained her birthweight and in spite of becoming ill several times and now relying on almost total ventilation, it was felt that she must have an operation to close her duct.

Rachel survived it remarkably well. But then she stopped passing urine. In 48 hours she went from 738g (1lb 10oz) to 915g (2lb) and our scrawny scrap of a daughter suddenly had a robust chest and a grotesque chin like a frog's. As a result of liquid retention, Rachel's potassium level had risen to a level which would kill an adult. It seemed that Rachel's kidneys had collapsed through the trauma of the operation. The doctors were prepared to do invasive dialysis, but we felt that our little daughter had been picked and squeezed, transfused, dripped so much that if life couldn't be sustained without this shock treatment, it was not worth sustaining. We wanted to let Rachel go before she lost her last vestige of dignity. It was agreed. That evening we installed ourselves in one of the parents' bedrooms and Rachel was brought to us in a shawl, already with very little life left in her. After Rachel had been confirmed dead, we bathed and dressed her in her first clothes, the smallest available hospital hand-me-downs, which were far too big for her.

A week later we held a funeral for Rachel which we think was a joyous event and of which we are quite proud. We then escaped to Norway: my cousin lent us a log cabin beside a lake and far from civilisation. At 37, with one miscarriage and one neonatal death behind me, I am not very close to my lifelong wish to have children, but I have hope and a good husband.

An account of the funeral Sue and Chris arranged for Rachel appears in chapter 6. This can be a difficult area, and one that has to be faced when parents are often at their most vulnerable. That chapter also gives examples of Rachel's birth and death announcements, sent to relatives and friends – another point of difficulty for many parents – which may perhaps be helpful for people who do not know how to respond to the situation.

Trisomy 13

Like Trisomy 18, Trisomy 13 or Patau's syndrome (formerly known as D Trisomy) is caused by an extra chromosome – this time number 13. More families have been affected by Trisomies 13 and 18 than is realised. Up to 50 per cent of pregnancies miscarry within days of conception, and one in five confirmed pregnancies ends naturally before twelve weeks: a high proportion of these spontaneous losses are believed to be chromosomally abnormal. Babies born with Trisomy 13 often need the intensive care that only a hospital or hospice can provide, but some infants are well enough to be nursed at home by loving parents. Equal numbers of boys and girls are born with Trisomy 13 and account for approximately one in 4,000 total births. The knowledge that a baby is affected by one of these conditions has a traumatic and immediate effect on families.

Helen
After a couple of scares in early pregnancy my antenatal visits proceeded normally, although my 'bump' never grew particularly large. However, when I visited the consultant the second time he was concerned about my size and a scan confirmed his fears. My longed-for first baby was severely growth retarded. Although I was 27 weeks pregnant, 'junior' only measured around 20 weeks.

I was told that my baby was dying, he was in severe distress, something had gone terribly wrong and I must wait for him to die before I could deliver him. Two weeks later I delivered my stillborn son. I can't tell you how bad those two weeks were for us. We were stuck in limbo, in the middle of some terrible nightmare that part of me was sure couldn't be happening to us.

My son's death was due to a chromosomal abnormality, Trisomy 13, which explained his slow development in the womb. The subsequent wait for the results of our chromosome tests was extremely stressful. I was convinced we would be carriers of this syndrome. Fortunately, we are not. Almost immediately (two months afterwards), I became pregnant again but miscarried at seven weeks.

Since my son was born, it has been pretty hard dealing with all the emotions that go with it. I didn't know I could ever be so depressed. I get on with life, of course, but everything's changed. It's very hard to enjoy other people's happiness now. I feel sick when I hear of other women's pregnancies, sick with jealousy, yet I marvel that they seem to produce babies so easily; it seems almost an impossible task for me to achieve. I guess I do wallow in my misery a lot, but the only thing I can think of that will lessen the pain is to have a baby, a live one.

Down's syndrome

A child with Down's syndrome has an extra chromosome 21, resulting in a disruption to the growth of the developing body. This extra chromosome can come from either the mother or the father, and is present because of a genetic accident when the egg or the sperm is produced, or during the initial cell division. Some 95 per cent of people with Down's syndrome have standard Trisomy 21, which always occurs because of such an 'accident of nature'. It can happen to anyone and there is no known reason why it occurs. The other 5 per cent may have inherited the condition from one of their parents because of a genetic abnormality called a translocation. It is known that the chances of parents of one child with Down's syndrome having a second child with the condition can be greater than that of the general population. Genetic counselling is therefore very important.

Many parents record the intense happiness and wonder which their Down's syndrome children have brought to their lives. These children are, on the whole, joyful and delightful beings. However, Down's syndrome brings with it a number of associated physical problems, such as congenital deafness, heart disease, leukaemia and intestinal narrowing. Many parents feel that they are unable to cope with the risk of increased suffering this may cause their child, or the disruption to family life. Bonnie writes for us here, recording her pain and loss.

Bonnie
I was so thrilled to be pregnant. I had a four-year-old son from a previous relationship, whom I love dearly, but was so excited to be expecting a baby with the man I loved. However, from the very beginning I wondered why I felt so ill, not just the usual sickness or exhaustion. I was in pain, but was continuously reassured that there was nothing wrong. So why did I need to return to hospital for so many scans? It would have been better to have been told from the beginning the possibility of there being something wrong. Instead, I was left with my mind swimming in a pool of frenzied suspicions.

At 19 weeks I was sent for yet another scan. I could not control my fears any longer. As the radiographer tapped away at the ultrasound machine, I cried and pleaded, 'What's wrong?' She would not tell me anything, but in her unwillingness to tell me what was going on inside my own body, with my own baby, I knew that there was something wrong. I had to wait to see the doctor. At last I was told. There was a tiny amount of fluid around the baby's heart. I was referred to another hospital to confirm the findings. It was then that I was informed I was carrying a baby girl, and I was reassured there was nothing to worry about. That made all the months of pain worthwhile. Of course every expectant mother just wants a healthy baby, but as my first baby was a son, a girl was the icing on the cake. It all seemed too good to be true. But the thrill of it all was like morphine for the pain which had become a normal part of this pregnancy.

At 25 weeks I collapsed and was taken to hospital. I had a scan taken at 26 weeks. The fluid was still around the baby's heart. I wanted to know the consequences of this. Another scan at 27 weeks showed the fluid had increased. It was bizarre that despite all this, and the fact that I had been in constant pain, I was still being reassured by the hospital.

At 28 weeks a foetal blood test was taken. I cried continuously as I awaited the result. My mind rolled over the ocean of possibilities: anaemia, cleft palate, hole in the heart, etc. Eventually the phone rang. My doctor asked if my husband was with me; he wasn't, but I still demanded to know whatever it was that he didn't want to tell me. There was a heavy silence followed by the shattering news that I was carrying a Down's syndrome baby, a very poorly little girl. She was probably very seriously retarded and wasn't expected to live long after birth. I was alive but dead. I was 29 weeks pregnant. All along, I had wanted to know what was going on inside my body. I felt I had been taken over by machines, monitors, medical terminology. Now the ball was thrown full force into my court as I helplessly made the decision, not lightly, to have a termination. How could I carry on my pregnancy to have her whisked away to tubes, operations, pain and then hand her over to death? How could I let her suffer further? It was the hardest decision I had ever had to make in my life.

Whatever I did or did not do, my baby was going to die. Some people will think I took an easy option. There was no easy option. My termination was not to involve an unwanted 'blob', the result of an 'accident'. I had created something out of love, a baby whom I already adored and desired more than anything else in the world. I had to go through labour to deliver my dead daughter. I was put on a drip and was given an epidural.

At 1.57am on Sunday 30 August, my darling Sian Alisa was born. I felt comforted that she was born on Sunday, a holy day. Perhaps God had wanted her from the beginning. I delivered her into death, not life, but I delivered her into peace, not pain. I held her tiny 2lb (0.9kg) body, so fragile, so delicate. She looked beautiful. I cuddled her, I kissed her and I told her how much Mummy loved her and how much she always will. How sorry I was for any pain she'd suffered. Life seemed so cruel. It was like staring at a treasured gift I knew I could not keep.

I insisted on getting my Sian baptised. I'll never forget how beautiful and peaceful she looked. It is ironic that Sian never had a certificate of birth, only of death. She was born with a translocation of her chromosomes, which meant she was severely retarded. Her heart and lungs would have given in.

I was put in a ward among all the mothers and their new babies. I had nothing, just total emptiness. My body ached all over. My eyes were red and so sore from my endless tears. No one could fully understand and no one could help. I live in silent sadness now because people cannot talk about it with me – perhaps they don't want to or think I don't want to. But I don't want Sian to be forgotten. When programmes crop up on TV about child loss, the people in the room grow silent and can't bear for their eyes to meet mine. Everyone's heart goes out to me but no words are spoken.

Of course, life goes on. Later I had another baby. Again, this pregnancy was not without its severe complications but, thankfully, I now have two adorable sons. They bring me much comfort and happiness. However, in my moments of happiness I think of Sian. I will make sure that her brothers know her. My eyes treasure my two little photographs of her, but as I am now divorced and her father has left me, I remember alone. I have learnt to cope and rebuild my life, but her memory still brings tears to my eyes and aches to my heart. I held her for such a little while.

Heart defects

Any expectant mother can tell of a whole host of frightening possibilities, the risk of problems for her precious child. It is certainly true that there is an endless list of potential congenital abnormalities, and it would be medically impossible for antenatal care to check for them all.

Heart defects are a case in point. From the twenty-fourth week of pregnancy onwards the foetal heart can be heard with a stethoscope, and from as early as the twelfth week it may be listened to with the use of a Sonicaid. Furthermore, ultrasound scans will demonstrate movement of the foetal heart as early as the end of the sixth week of pregnancy.

During a 'normal' pregnancy, the baby's heart will be checked visually once, or possibly twice, at ultrasound scans, and checked audibly at each regular antenatal appointment. There are many possible heart defects, however, which cannot be diagnosed through these methods, and so it is still all too possible for major heart defects to go undiagnosed.

The shock of discovering that a baby, believed throughout the pregnancy to be perfect, is fatally ill is portrayed here for us by Angela. Her words bring home the trauma of such sudden realisation.

Angela

The first time I became pregnant I miscarried at 13 weeks. It was devastating and I felt that no one understood my grief – everyone seemed to think that 'we were young and could try again'. My gynaecologist told me that there was no investigation into the causes of miscarriage until 'you've had at least three'.

I became pregnant again six months later – I needed some help in early pregnancy when I threatened to miscarry again, but luckily carried my baby to term and our daughter, Laura, was born to our great joy. I became pregnant again after trying for a while, had problems at the beginning of the pregnancy but carried the baby to term and our second daughter, Alexia, was born.

Unfortunately, our happiness was shortlived as unbeknown to us she was suffering from a major heart defect and had breathing problems as soon as she was born – I held her in my arms for two minutes and then she was whisked away to intensive care. She died the next day. My husband and I were devastated and I sincerely think that no one can understand how you feel unless they have been in that situation themselves. The worst thing in the world must surely be going to your own child's funeral. I still have nightmares about it.

Afterwards, I felt extremely isolated. In fact I still find it extremely difficult to talk about it five years later, and occasionally a feeling of loss will flood over me and I find myself in tears. I had to find my own way out of this black hole of despair and realised that if I didn't make an effort I would just go mad and make life hell for my husband and other daughter. I looked into prams all the time and imagined what my little baby would be like if she had lived. I can sincerely understand women who are so desperate that they take someone else's baby even if they know that it is wrong.

Luckily, my story has a happy ending as we had another daughter, our little Jessica. I had to undergo fertility treatment and then endure nine months of anxiety, but I now look back on all those years when I was trying to have my family as a real wilderness.

Spina bifida and hydrocephalus

Spina bifida is a fault in the spinal column in which one or more vertebrae fail to form properly, leaving a gap or split. It is one of the most common defects present at birth in Britain, although the incidence varies from one geographical area to another. The Association for Spina Bifida and Hydrocephalus (ASBAH) produces an excellent booklet detailing the medical technicalities, which are not strictly relevant to this book.

At present, the cause of spina bifida is unknown (it is thought to be connected with both genetic and environmental factors), and therefore prevention is not always possible, although research continues and certain preventive measures are currently recommended. Doctors now believe that folic acid taken before conception and during the first 12–14 weeks of pregnancy may help to prevent the occurrence of the condition. This advice springs from a large-scale study published in 1991 which showed that large doses of folic acid can be crucial in preventing the recurrence of neural tube defects. The recommendations are that pregnant women with no history of spina bifida should take 400 micrograms (mcg) of folic acid (available over the counter at chemists), and that vulnerable women should take 5 milligrams (mg), via a doctor's prescription.

Spina bifida is only partly hereditary. However, if parents have one sufferer in the family, there is an increased risk of another child being born with it too. Genetic counselling is available for parents who are known to be at risk. Sherry tells now of the heartbreak involved in such cases.

Sherry
On 15 February our first child, Sarah Anne Louise, was born. She was a very much wanted and planned baby. Although I suffered

terrible morning sickness for the first three months, the rest of my pregnancy progressed normally. At 20 weeks, blood was taken for a test which I was told would detect spina bifida and Down's syndrome. I was very relieved when the results were returned and appeared normal. I still worried, as all mothers-to-be do, and had an awful gut feeling that there would be no baby at the end of my pregnancy.

Later, as I was a few days overdue and my blood pressure had started to go up, I was admitted to hospital and induced the following morning. Labour began quickly and strongly and by lunchtime I was told I might need a forceps delivery as the head was quite large. I was determined to try on my own and managed after only a couple of pushes. It was then that the atmosphere in the labour ward changed dramatically and I knew my worst fears had come true – something was wrong. All eyes fell to the floor and when I asked what was wrong, at first no one answered. Sarah was crying and my husband, Geoff, said, 'Don't worry, she's crying loudly, everything is OK.' I cried out, 'What is the matter? Tell me.' It was a moment Geoff and I will never forget, and it is as vivid now as it was 15 years ago. The paediatrician came over and held both my hands in his and said, 'Sherry, you must be very brave – there is a hole in her spinal cord.' I screamed, 'Spina bifida,' and Geoff fell to the floor. He couldn't believe it as Sarah weighed over 8lbs (3.6kg) and looked so beautiful.

I was given a sedative straight away and then did something I will regret for the rest of my life – when the nurse brought Sarah over to me I could not take her. I don't know why. I felt anger, disappointment, guilt, bitterness – so many emotions took over at once. Sarah was taken to the Special Care Unit, and I was taken to the isolation ward so that I was not among the new mothers and their healthy babies. I cannot praise the hospital staff enough for their care before, during and after Sarah's birth and death.

The following days and weeks were as if it was all a dream. Sarah was assessed by a leading authority on spina bifida. She had a lesion which covered 60 per cent of her back. She also had hydrocephalus (water on the brain), which accounted for her unusually large head. We were told that the doctors draw an imaginary line to assess these cases; babies above this line can be helped and given a certain quality of life, but babies below this line have no hope of a reasonable quality of life and would have to endure endless operations each year to be kept alive. Sarah was well below the line.

There was no decision to be taken in our view and the doctors agreed. We both felt that in this world you need to be 100 per cent fit to cope, and that brain damage and major physical problems could not be overcome. I know that this is not a view held by everyone, but it was our baby and our decision. I would never want to influence other people in this situation as it is up to each person to make their own decisions.

Sarah was demand-fed by nurses, but her back and her hydrocephalus were not treated. It took nearly seven weeks for her to die. I kept asking why she couldn't be allowed to die with dignity and why they couldn't give her something to ease her suffering. We watched her grow weaker and weaker and gradually go into a coma. The doctors insisted that I should look at her problems, because if I did not then after her death I might not believe how ill she really had been. One of her legs had not developed properly and was small and twisted. That was awful to see, but the worst was that her bottom was not properly developed along with the spinal cord. When she was dressed and wrapped up she looked so beautiful.

We were encouraged not to visit her too much as getting too attached would make it even harder at the end. We both appreciated and understood this advice, but as the weeks went on we visited her more and more and took her flowers from our garden and small gifts. Eventually she slipped away one Saturday morning. We went to say goodbye to Sarah that afternoon and although I had seen my mother after her death, I was not prepared to see our beautiful daughter so pale and still. The vividness of these memories is still with me and I am sure they will never fade.

We decided not to try straight away for another child, but to get advice on the odds of it happening again and any preventive measures we could take to try to stop it.

The doctors explained that the blood test had given a false negative result and because of this, and a few other similar mistakes, the test was now only to be given at 16 weeks of pregnancy to give a more accurate result.

I eventually became pregnant again and had a blood test and amniocentesis. Waiting for the results were the longest three weeks of my life, but they came out clear and I gave birth to another girl, Louise Elizabeth. We had doctors standing by to check her the moment she was born, and words cannot express our relief and joy when we were told she was OK. I fed her immediately and never even felt the stitches the doctor put in. I was on cloud nine.

When Louise was two years old we began thinking that a brother or sister would be good for her. We were not as worried as before; having one healthy baby had given us a real boost.

Our third baby girl was due in June, and again I had the blood test and amniocentesis at 16 weeks. Being busy with a two-year-old, the three weeks' wait passed a lot quicker this time. The specialist was lovely and kind, but I can still hear his words: 'I am so sorry, Sherry, it has happened again ...' The amnio and subsequent scan showed another badly affected baby. I was nearly 20 weeks pregnant by this time and could feel the baby moving. We both knew there was no point in going any further with the pregnancy and I was admitted the following morning to have the pregnancy terminated. Abortion seems such a hard word to me, and I still shudder when I hear it. Labour had to be induced, but mercifully it did not take too long. I sent Geoff home just before the end with the excuse that Louise needed him. I did not look at the baby when it was delivered and I do not regret that decision at all. I was given a D&C the following morning and went home that evening. Again, the staff were marvellous and could not have been kinder to us.

I felt relieved that we had not gone a full nine months only to lose our baby again, but I was not prepared for the shock to my system after the termination. I have never regretted it, since we knew it was the best for all of us – the baby, Louise, Geoff and myself – but to be pregnant one minute and not the next has a very odd effect on your body. It took some weeks for my body to realise there was no baby and my hormones to return to normal.

We went back to see the specialist and ask his advice about trying one more time for a baby. He was really super and said that at least I was able to conceive easily, which was more than a lot of people could do. He said if he was in our situation he would have one more go. This time I had to take multivitamins with folic acid for at least three months before trying again. This I did and conceived a beautiful healthy baby boy (Ross Alexander). What a fantastic Christmas we had that year.

We consider ourselves to be a very fortunate family and of course all life is precious, but Louise and Ross are really extra special.

I consider we had expert help and support from all the staff at the hospital, and we owe our healthy family to them.

I remember taking part in a college debate against abortion when only 16 years old. Never had I thought that one day I might need one. My experiences have certainly taught me never to prejudge a situation and say how one would react, because unless you are faced with it personally you just never know.

Hydrocephalus is commonly, but inaccurately, known as 'water on the brain'. A watery fluid is produced constantly inside each of the four ventricles inside the brain. It normally flows through narrow pathways, out over the inside of the brain and down the spinal cord. If the drainage pathways are obstructed at any point, the fluid accumulates inside the brain, causing the ventricles to swell and resulting in compression of the surrounding tissue. In babies and infants the head will enlarge, but this is not possible in older children and adults, since the bones of the skull are then completely joined.

Babies delivered prematurely are at risk of developing hydrocephalus, mainly because the blood vessels in the brain are very fragile and can easily burst, putting the baby at risk of a haemorrhage which in turn can produce a blood clot big enough to break through the wall of the ventricle, blocking the flow of the cerebro-spinal fluid.

Most babies born with spina bifida have hydrocephalus, allied to abnormalities in the physical structure of certain parts of the brain which develop before birth. This prevents proper drainage of the fluid from the brain.

Hydrocephalus can also be caused by a brain haemorrhage, meningitis or a tumour. In extremely rare circumstances, it can be hereditary.

Some forms of hydrocephalus require no specific treatment. Other forms are temporary and do not require long-term treatment. Most forms, however, do require treatment, usually the surgical implant of a shunting device which diverts accumulated fluid, thus preventing the condition from becoming worse. Symptoms caused by raised pressure usually improve but other problems of brain damage will remain.

The result is that babies born with hydrocephalus (and spina bifida), who 30 years ago would probably have died, now have a dramatically improved life expectancy. However, too many die still.

ASBAH plays a leading role in the support for families of children suffering from these illnesses. Its address can be found in chapter 8.

The parents who have contributed to this chapter have shared their raw emotions in order to help provide knowledge to those who must follow. We cannot thank them enough for sharing their deepest thoughts, so that future sufferers need not feel quite so alone.

4 What if there is no reason or cause?

People are all different; we are all unique, and will respond to losing a baby in a variety of ways. Some parents can cry immediately, while others find the reality hits them later. Some need to talk to anyone who will listen, but especially an empathetic person, while others will wish to immerse themselves in their day-to-day responsibilities to keep themselves occupied. Some parents need to find a cause, a reason, perhaps something to blame; others may be more philosophical in accepting life's uncertainties.

A number of parents will wish to find out as much as possible about their baby's condition and thus try to understand why the death occurred. Many parents find that a post-mortem result is in some way comforting; it may extricate them from guilt feelings that their actions may have harmed the baby in some way, or it may mean that they can begin to explain to others in terms of certainty what happened in their case. A parent's distress may, however, be exacerbated if the post-mortem finds no physiological reason for the cause of death. Parents may be left with doubts, perhaps guilt feelings, not because they did anything wrong but because they don't know if there was something they could have done to prevent the death. It is the not knowing which deepens the pain still further. Some will understandably, want to find a target to blame. In many cases, this may be the medical staff who dealt with the delivery. It is easy to forget that medical staff are human and may sometimes make errors, and that technology is not always 100 per cent reliable, but this is easy to say if it is not your baby who has died. When we hand ourselves, our bodies and our babies over to medical experts, we expect that things should go well – it surely must be the case that most medical practitioners wish they had the power to ensure that. However, it must be said that in the small number of cases where the evidence suggests that the medical profession were at fault, doctors are doing parents a disservice by not accepting blame where it is due.

Anita is a parent who sadly lost her son, Alexander, for what seemed to be no reason. A highly educated woman, with a medical background, she was keen to see the post-mortem results, as she believed that having a reason for her son's death would make it easier to accept. Only a few days before the birth, Anita's son had been alive. She feels that she was not given adequate care when she visited the hospital and that subsequent discussions with the consultant were also less than helpful – indeed, the circumstances were distressing – although she praises the work of the midwives.

Anita

Just over eight weeks ago, our long-awaited first child, Alexander, was stillborn at 39 weeks in the maternity department of our local teaching hospital. Towards the end of my pregnancy, I was diagnosed as having high blood pressure. As a consequence of this, I was admitted to hospital twice for observation, the first time for 48 hours and on the second occasion for 24 hours. On my second admission, the doctor in charge arranged an induction date for me, 21 June, which was, in her words, 'unfortunately the earliest date available', presumably due to financial constraints.

On Friday 18 June I attended the day assessment unit, where my blood pressure and urine were checked. I was then attached to a monitor to determine the wellbeing of my baby. The machine continued to monitor me for over one hour, instead of the usual 20 minutes, and both the doctor and midwife attending me seemed unsure as to how to interpret the trace which was obtained. I was asked whether I had been drinking coffee, as my baby's heartrate appeared to be accelerated. We were assured, however, that there were no problems: the results obtained were most likely attributable to the baby being asleep and the reduction in movements that I had described were 'normal' at this late stage.

On Monday 21 June I was admitted to hospital in my thirty-ninth week of pregnancy for an induction. The midwife attending me could not find our baby's heartbeat. The fact that our son had died was confirmed by an ultrasound scan which showed his heart had stopped beating. I was then told by the doctor and midwives attending me that although our baby was dead, I would have to deliver him normally. They were unwilling to perform a Caesarean section due to possible scarring to my womb which might complicate future pregnancies. They also explained that psychologically it was the best way, as I would then realise that I had given birth and that my baby had died.

The night of 21 June was the worst of my life and I only got through it because my husband was with me all the time. The next morning we were taken down to the delivery suite. After a long labour, during which we were supported by the midwives, our family and close friends, our beautiful son, Alexander, was born at 11.10pm. It was desperately sad but also a wonderful moment for us when we saw him and held him just after he was born. The following day, he was brought to us and we had him blessed and took some photographs. My mum and two of our close friends also held our baby. It seems so pathetic now that while other parents have their babies to hold and love, all we have is a lock of our baby's hair, his hand- and footprints and some photographs. They are not much, but they are a great comfort to us.

Two weeks ago, we met with the consultant to discuss the results of the post-mortem and also of tests which were performed on me to determine the cause of death. We felt that day would be a turning point for us, since we would find out why our baby died and this would make it easier to accept. The post-mortem confirmed that our baby had no abnormalities and, the tests performed on me were also negative. The consultant conceded that if our son had been induced even a few days earlier he would, as we had suspected, almost certainly be alive. In addition, on examining the trace of our baby's heart activity which was obtained at the day assessment unit on 18 June, he accepted it did not look normal. He is currently determining whether the trace was indicating that our baby was in distress on that day.

In the immediate aftermath of the discovery of Alexander's death, my own community midwife, my GP and the midwifery staff at the hospital were all extremely supportive to my husband and myself. Their consideration for our feelings, however, stands in stark contrast to the treatment we received when we visited the consultant to discuss the stillbirth. On this occasion, we were asked to attend a regular gynaecological clinic where we had to wait almost one hour among many pregnant women with small children. We found this treatment extremely insensitive, to say the least. Our region has few stillbirths each year; it would not seem to be beyond the capabilities of the department concerned to arrange for bereaved parents such as ourselves to be seen at a separate time and place. As it was, all the good work and counselling of the midwives was completely undermined by our treatment at that clinic.

We now find it very difficult to come to terms with the death of our baby since we feel that it happened needlessly. We have not received an official apology or an explanation from the hospital concerning the unusual circumstances of our perfectly normal baby's death. All they can say is that next time they will look after me very carefully. Well, why couldn't they have done so this time?

Explanations and redress

Medicine is not an exact science and mistakes may be made, some of which may have devastating consequences. In a situation like Anita's, you might want simply to find out more about what went wrong, or you might want legal redress.

Before making any kind of legal complaint, it may be useful to ask the medical personnel involved for more information and to offer them a chance to give an explanation.

The big problem with any complaint about medical treatment is that many matters come down to a question of clinical judgement, which is not usually a black-and-white, clear-cut issue. The complaint is likely to centre on questions of negligence, perhaps due to poor staffing levels, which you may feel have contributed to the problem. A hospital is under a duty to provide care and treatment of a reasonable standard. Poor staffing levels do not dilute the nature of that duty. If a patient suffers adverse consequences because he or she has been unable to see a midwife or doctor, for example (because there aren't enough on duty), the hospital may be liable for negligence (see below).

To complain about treatment there are various steps to follow, First, raise the issue informally with your consultant. If you are not satisfied with the outcome, write to the hospital complaints officer, who will refer the matter to the Regional Medical Officer (RMO). The RMO may decide to set up an independent professional review for a serious complaint, but may only agree to start this procedure if you agree not to take any legal action about your complaint. This is not usually legally binding, but at this stage you may wish to take advice from your solicitor or Community Health Council (CHC).

If you want an explanation, rather than redress, this may be the best course of action. Under the review procedure, your case will be considered by two independent consultants currently practising in the relevant specialist area. If they find the treatment was correct, they will then discuss it further with you; if not, they will discuss it with the medical staff concerned. They then report their findings and you will eventually receive a letter explaining the outcome.

If you are unhappy with this, you may decide to contact your CHC, although there is no right of appeal. The Health Service Ombudsman may be able to help if you feel the complaint was not properly handled, but more often than not such problems will fall outside the ombudsman's jurisdiction.

If you feel that the treatment you received resulted in you suffering pain, injury or inconvenience, this may amount to negligence and if so, you may wish to claim compensation.

Interestingly, while a number of parents who contributed to this book wanted explanations, no one mentioned legal redress and action for negligence. This may be because the contributors did not feel negligence applied in their cases, or perhaps because medical negligence is a legal minefield which people in the UK tend to avoid.

Negligence

Professional negligence is where a practitioner does not provide care of a standard usually provided by a competent practitioner, or makes a mistake which a competent practitioner would not make. All patients have a legal right to be treated with reasonable care and reasonable skill. The way this is judged is in relation to other members of the profession – what would they have done in the same circumstances? In treating you, your doctor therefore undertakes to have the same skill level as the average, reasonable doctor.

If you feel you are entitled to compensation as a result of negligence, you are in a complex situation and need to consult a solicitor. It really is essential to consult a solicitor with experience and training in medical negligence, and many firms of solicitors will not be suitable for such a claim. Your local Citizens' Advice Bureau may be able to assist you in finding an appropriate solicitor. The onus of proof is on you, the patient, to prove that the practitioner failed to act with reasonable care and so failed to meet the standard of competence compatible with his/her training and experience – for this you will need expert help.

Legal action for negligence must usually be started within three years of the injury or damage. However, where a child is involved, the three-year time limit for making a claim only applies once he or she reaches 18 years of age; while in respect of a claim for a mentally handicapped person, it does not apply at all as long as that person is incapable of managing his or her affairs. Nevertheless, if legal action is to be considered, consult a solicitor as soon as is reasonably practicable.

These facts may be particularly pertinent in cases of cerebral palsy, where a significant number of cases are caused by birth asphyxia which should have been avoided.

You can take court action even if you are simultaneously taking a complaint through other channels, but if this is the case any health authority investigation will be suspended until the outcome of the legal action is known.

It is worth being aware that medical negligence cases can be messy, long and expensive, but they are an option if you feel there is a case to answer. The first steps a solicitor will take will be to obtain copies of the relevant medical records and then to seek opinions from medical experts from the field in which negligence is suspected. Legal Aid may be available to assist with legal costs, and is nearly always available for legal action on behalf of a child, provided there is a prima facie case.

Conversely, taking such action may prolong the period of grieving felt by any parent who loses a baby before, at or soon after birth.

Four years before she contacted us, Jacquie lost her baby son for seemingly no reason. He was a good birthweight, and the only possible warning sign she noticed was a decrease in movements at the end of an uneventful pregnancy. However, this is common in most pregnancies as the growing baby becomes more confined within the womb, and many people would not be too worried about this. The post-mortem on Daniel gave no cause for his death, but Jacquie actually found this somehow comforting. She felt that she could not blame herself or anyone else, because there was nothing she or they could have done until it was too late. In some ways, this may be easier to come to terms with than the recriminations which may be felt if the finger of blame is pointed by a post-mortem. We hope that Jacquie's report is helpful to newly bereaved parents, because she has had four years to come to terms with her loss and her story illustrates that for many people the pain does become more manageable in time.

Jacquie
It's four years ago that my baby son was stillborn. I still miss him very much, but the pain is far less. If any part of my story is of help to others, I shall feel there was some significance to his little life. I had a very uneventful pregnancy and had reached the last days. My baby was due on Monday, but on Sunday I began to worry because there didn't seem to be as much movement as usual. By the middle of the night, I began to get frightened, but with our three-year-old asleep in the other room I didn't think there was much I could do until morning. My husband, Brian, obviously sensed my concern and didn't leave for work before I made the call to the hospital. The voice at the other end of the phone had a calm urgency: 'Come in at once.'

We were taken straight to a room where we waited for what seemed ages, but was probably only minutes. When the midwife came with a foetal monitor, she couldn't find a heartbeat and suggested I should have a scan. The scan confirmed my fears – my baby had died. I was completely numb. I couldn't cry, especially not in front of others. Brian and I were taken to a little room and left on our own. I think it was felt we needed time to come to terms with what had happened. I really just wanted someone to tell me what would happen next and just take over for me – I didn't want to think or make decisions. Eventually a doctor came to talk to us. He said I'd have to have labour induced and as my first labour had been long, I should expect this one to take a long time. He then said I could choose when to have this done: I could come in there and then, although they were very busy that day, or I could come in the next day, or Wednesday would be best for them. But it was my decision; whatever I wanted to do, they'd do. He then left us to talk about it. I couldn't face a long wait; I wanted to get it all over with now. After a very short, sharp and uneventful labour, Daniel was born at 5.45pm weighing 9lb 15oz (4.52kg) and looking beautiful. The staff were all very nice and kind, but because they were so busy they couldn't give us the time they felt we needed. We didn't mind. By now my midwife who had seen me right through my pregnancy had arrived and gave us lots of advice.

It was on her advice that we cuddled our baby – for over an hour. That was so special. After months of waiting for him, as I cuddled him all the love I'd been waiting to pour out on him could well up and I could grieve for a real baby. Also, on our midwife's advice, we had Daniel's photo taken. It was on a polaroid camera and didn't really show how beautiful he was, but it's all I have of him and it's precious. I only wish I'd been advised to bring our own camera in with us. After all, it was ready in the hall, with everything else, just as it had been for days. But with the baby being dead, we never gave it a thought. A lot of the things our midwife said, we could have done with hearing hours earlier. Perhaps it was because they were so busy at the hospital that day.

Because the labour had been so quick, I hadn't had time to have the epidural I'd been advised to have (they said it couldn't harm the baby now, so I may as well have all the pain relief available) so my midwife persuaded the hospital to let me go home. Brian and I were sad to say goodbye to Daniel, but it was good to be in the privacy of our own home. That's when Brian wept. I woke in the night and was glad of Brian's arms to hold me as I sobbed and sobbed for my baby.

The days and weeks followed. I was exceptionally well looked after by my midwife and doctor. They took me through the discomfort of the milk coming in etc. that all had to be dealt with although the baby wasn't there. Family and friends were there when I needed them.

A post-mortem was carried out on Daniel, but no cause for his death was ever found. I found that a great comfort at the time – I couldn't blame myself or the professionals for anything we'd missed or not done. It had just been Daniel's time. I must admit that it wasn't too easy when I got pregnant again – I'd have loved to know what happened before, to be sure of avoiding it this time. Thankfully, my daughter arrived a year and one week later and is now a healthy girl of three. She'll never replace Daniel, but it's strange to think that if he hadn't died, she may never have lived.

From Anita's and Jacquie's reports, it becomes clear that women who are told their babies have died in the womb are not sure what to expect and often do not anticipate having to go through labour as they would had the baby been alive. This comes as something of a shock in many cases, but is seen to be psychologically beneficial so that the parents are aware of what has happened and can begin to grieve as they need to.

Another point which is commonly made in these contributions is that the mothers experienced a feeling of anxiety about the welfare of their babies, or noticed a decrease in movements. Any such anxieties should be reported to the hospital, which has the equipment to check the situation and perhaps help if there is still time; medical staff should never ignore such anxieties. Sometimes intuition and instinct can be reliable indicators of a problem.

The following report was written by a mother who discovered her baby had died in the womb, probably due to placental failure, although this was not certain from the post-mortem. It is easy in these circumstances to feel a sense of guilt that the baby's inactivity was not noted earlier, as this mother reveals, but she did in fact follow her instinctive feeling that something was wrong.

Anon

At 38 weeks gestation, I attended the hospital for my usual check-up. I was told everything was OK and to come back the following week. On the same night, I couldn't sleep because of the immense activity of my baby and I sat downstairs until it had settled. If only I had realised what was happening. The following day I went about my business as usual, thinking the baby was having a long lie.

Having felt no movement for a whole day, I called on my GP – he used his stethoscope and told me he could hear a heartbeat. Not convinced, I made my husband take me to the hospital. They attached me to a foetal monitor and were able to confirm my fears – there was no heartbeat. I was then admitted and given a date, three days later, for induction.

Two days later I was taken for an X-ray. I was escorted through the corridors alongside the baby wards and by the time I arrived for X-ray was in a rather distressed state. I was scolded by the female radiographer and told that my behaviour was not helping either me or the baby. I was then told to lie face down, which was difficult and uncomfortable. X-ray completed, I was returned to my room. Induction went ahead as planned.

They inserted a catheter smeared with something and, unknown to me, I went into labour during the night. I woke up with a sore back and sore legs, and the nurse gave me something to take away the pain. I was taken down to the labour ward in the morning for my promised epidural; however, the person who was to administer this was in theatre and by the time he was free, it was felt it was too late. Our daughter was born at lunchtime. The cord was wound tightly around her neck. The post-mortem revealed that there were no congenital or developmental abnormalities whatsoever and they suspected that death was due to placental failure.

I didn't wish to see the baby and then proceeded to bury my head in the sand. Obviously, both my husband and I grieved, but unfortunately not together. It was a taboo subject in the family as well, and three months later I was pregnant again. I have three children now, with a blighted pregnancy between numbers one and two.

On some occasions there is nothing physiologically wrong with the baby, but birth trauma can cause damage or even death. These days, most births tend to be less prolonged than they used to be and intervention is more frequent – involving induction, instrumental delivery or Caesarean section. Many question this trend, but in some ways it is inevitable that increased diagnostic skills and technology will lead to intervention to save the life of a baby. However, we still have reports where a birth did not go according to plan and where the baby was stillborn or died soon afterwards.

The following report from a contributor concerning the birth of her daughter, Miranda, is similar. Following an uneventful pregnancy, her baby daughter inhaled meconium (the black, sticky substance that babies usually pass from their bowels a few days after birth) and later died after treatment in the Special Care Unit. In this report, however, the mother felt that no one was to blame and that the event was an unhappy accident.

Stephanie
When I first heard that my baby was due on 14 February, I was delighted. We already had two sons, aged two and four, so, dare I admit it, I was secretly hoping that our third child would be a girl.

The months passed. I had a normal and easy pregnancy and the thought of the new baby kept us going as the dreary winter evenings grew longer and longer. Then 14 February arrived. I was playing with my two boys after tea when I first felt the pangs of labour. It was on the way to the maternity hospital that we finally decided that if it was a girl, we would call her Miranda. Labour was quick and easy and I managed without the help of painkilling drugs. Just before midnight, my baby daughter was delivered. She was beautiful, perfect, and I can say without question that it was the happiest moment of my life. In fact I was so elated that I hardly registered the midwife calling out, 'Bleep for a paediatrician, quick!' After ten minutes or so my daughter was given to me to hold, but only for a moment. She let out a tiny bleat like a little lamb and then they took her away.

The paediatrician explained that she had inhaled meconium, and that her lungs were clogged with it. He explained that they would try to pump out her lungs, but that she might be left with a tendency to coughs and respiratory infection. Gradually, as the night wore on, my supreme elation died away and a great dread and fear took hold of me. When the day staff came on duty I had to know what had happened, and I knew by the evasive answer, 'Your husband's coming,' that something very dreadful indeed had happened. When he arrived at about eight, he said that she was still alive but very seriously ill. In fact she was so ill that they had baptised her during the night, not expecting her to last until morning. We clung together and wept; it seemed so cruel that all our hopes should be dashed away overnight. The Sunday passed in a haze of comings and goings. People were so kind and I was surprised to find that the doctors and nurses were so upset.

We went to see her in the Special Care Baby Unit, a perfect baby but with her face horribly distorted by breathing tubes and her little chest heaving with every painful breath. Sunday night passed. I dared not sleep, terrified that if I did, she might die; I somehow thought that so long as I could keep awake I could will her to stay alive. On the Monday, at lunchtime, the consultant told us that both her lungs had punctured, and as the oxygen wasn't flowing properly around her body she might have suffered brain damage. We both knew that she was dying. We were back in the ward at teatime when the paediatrician came and told us that she had just passed away.

In a strange way, there was a sort of relief at the announcement; now at least we knew what we had to face. Later that evening we went to see her. She looked so utterly peaceful lying there motionless, compared with when we had last seen her, struggling for life amidst the noisy machinery and glaring lights of the Special Care Baby Unit, and I knew instantly that I was looking at a little glimpse of heaven. We held her in our arms. I only regret now that I didn't ask for her photograph, although her picture is of course forever engraved in my memory.

We decided to have her buried at home. Somehow in the numbness of shock in the days following her birth, it helped to have something to do, choosing the spot where she was to be buried in our quiet country churchyard, ordering flowers and so on. Everyone was very, very kind and we realised how lucky we were to live in a small village, in such a supportive community. But of course, it's difficult for people to know what to say and to understand what losing a baby can mean. I remember one well-meaning friend saying, 'How awful to go through nine months and end up with nothing.' But I hadn't ended up with nothing – I had ended up with a baby who had died, the most momentous experience of my life. I suppose that is one of the very cruel things about losing a baby at birth or soon after: you have so little to show for it – no photographs, no playschool paintings, no favourite teddies; you just come home from hospital to a house that to all outward appearances looks just as you had left it, except that the baby things have all been tactfully whisked away.

Life, of course, goes on. I never felt the slightest anger or bitterness; it seemed to me that since my baby had died it would be pointless to indulge in negative emotions that would never bring her back, but it was difficult, so difficult to accept that a perfect baby had to die, through an accident at birth.

For months, I veered wildly from living a normal, calm existence to moments of uncontrollable grief. Friends were wonderful. They listened for hour after hour. Talking about what had happened was what I needed to do, and I sought out new faces so that I could tell them. I once even told the girl at the supermarket checkout that my baby had died. Many people don't realise that some bereaved people have a burning need to talk, and fear they are upsetting you if you cry. In fact all that grief is bottled up inside you, so tears are a welcome relief.

The fact that I was pregnant again after six months didn't seem to help at all. I knew that friends and doctors secretly thought all would be well now that I was pregnant, but I only felt guilty and forlorn, because I truthfully didn't want another baby, only the same one back again. It was at this time that I joined my local SANDS. This I found an enormous support, and because everyone was in the same position we could exchange experiences without embarrassment.

In the years since my baby died I have had three more children (delivered by Caesarean section), all boys, so I never had much time to brood. I think I have a much clearer idea of what is really important than I have ever had before, and the gift of life has never seemed so precious. Nevertheless, when the children come running home from school on 14 February with their cards that they've made saying 'Happy Valentine's Day', I smart inwardly from a great, gaping wound that will never go away.

Meconium in the amniotic waters indicates problems and hospital staff take it very seriously. In many cases it is a sign of foetal distress, so delivery of the baby is then expedited – it may cause no problems other than an accelerated labour. It cannot be anticipated in advance, but is something which is noted during labour. Likewise, the baby's heartbeat is usually monitored carefully, sometimes by listening through the mother's abdomen at regular intervals if all seems well, or by continuous electronic monitoring through an electrode attached to the baby's head if the labour is prolonged or difficult or there are signs of problems.

The following report details the birth and death of this mother's son, Adam, who was a perfectly healthy baby until distress during labour, when he was deprived of oxygen, which caused fatal brain damage. This mother's bitter response is very natural, given a healthy pregnancy and the shock of her loss.

Hayley

My husband and I had been married for 18 months when I found that I was pregnant. I went for a scan at 18 weeks and everything seemed fine. We went along to parentcraft classes and were beginning to get excited about the birth of our much-wanted baby. The baby was due on 25 February, so when I got to 10 March and still nothing had happened, I was beginning to get a bit fed up. My doctor said he would give me another week before sending me to be induced. The following day I stayed in bed, as I wasn't feeling too good. Later I had a show, so I telephoned the delivery suite and they said I was probably in early labour. They asked if the baby still seemed active, and when I replied 'No,' they asked me in. When the doctor examined me, he said he felt that 15 days overdue was enough and they would induce me at 6 o'clock the following morning. Although I was a little nervous, I was relieved that the waiting would finally be over.

I was induced early in the morning, but for the first hour or so nothing seemed to happen. Then I gradually started to feel contractions quite regularly. I was put on a monitor to check the baby's heartrate and all seemed to be fine. At 8am my husband arrived, equipped with a camera ready for the occasion. It seemed to be a long morning. I got in and out of the bath three times, as the midwife said it was best to keep active in the first stage of labour. At 10 o'clock she examined me to see if I was dilating, and said she could feel the top of our baby's head and could feel some hair. We were both so excited. She then injected some more prostogen gel to speed things up. By 12.30 I was having contractions every five minutes and they were becoming unbearable, so the midwife decided to move me back to the delivery suite. I tried to manage with gas and oxygen because I wanted as natural a birth as possible, but the pain became too much at about 1.45 and I was given pethidine, which was marvellous. I seemed to sleep for the next hour. Then, slowly, the pain began to come back.

At about 3pm I went to the toilet and thought my waters had broken because I felt a gush from inside, but it was actually my baby messing inside me. Still, nobody seemed to be worried. I then had to have my waters broken, and I had dilated to 4 centimetres. I was put back on the monitor, as the midwife was having trouble hearing the heartbeat through the handheld instrument. Our baby's heartbeat was becoming very erratic, so they decided to attach a probe to his head to get a better reading. At this stage, the doctor decided to give me an epidural as he thought it was going to be a long night and I needed to keep my strength up. By this time, our baby's heartbeat kept dropping rapidly and then coming back up. My husband and I were beginning to get worried, but we knew we were in safe hands. By 6pm they decided to take a blood sample from my baby's head, and from that moment it was all systems go. I was rushed for an emergency Caesarean and although I was nervous, I still did not think anything could go wrong.

At 6.40 on the evening of 12 March, our beautiful son, Adam, was born. He weighed 7lb 1oz (3.21kg) and was barely breathing. He was taken straight to SCBU.

That night, all I can remember is my husband saying we had a son and he showed me a photo that had been taken in SCBU, but I was still under anaesthetic and was not really with it. It wasn't until the following morning that I realised how seriously ill our son was.

We saw the doctor in SCBU and he told us that Adam had been starved of oxygen during labour; they did not know the extent of the damage, but it did not look too good. He was fitting all the time and he was very limp. When I saw him for the first time, he had tubes coming out of everywhere and he was also on a ventilator to help him breathe. I was numb and could not believe what was happening.

We had a glimmer of hope when Adam was five days old when he came off his ventilator, but 24 hours later he started fitting again. The doctors did not think Adam would be able to live without the aid of a ventilator. They said it would be best to leave it off and let Adam decide whether or not he would pull through.

At 2.45am on 18 March our precious son, Adam, died in my arms. Although I would not have wanted him to suffer, I felt very bitter that this had happened to us. A post-mortem showed that Adam was a healthy baby until he got into distress in labour. I would like people to know that things don't always go smoothly when having a baby, because when you read all the baby books they seem to make things look rosy. My husband and I would never have dreamt that this could happen to us.

It is over a year now since we lost Adam and we visit his grave every week. I don't think you ever get over the loss of a child, but you do learn to live with your feelings. You just have to take one day at a time. I have helped to form a self-help group, which has helped me to survive the black days. I find it important to talk about Adam, because he was a major part of our life and always will be.

A happy footnote – Hayley and her husband now have a beautiful, healthy daughter, Danielle.

Even during a straightforward delivery, the experience of birth is quite a traumatic one for a baby. After nine months or so in the womb, warm and safe, he or she is suddenly pushed quite violently through the narrow tunnel of the cervix and vagina, into the outside world. Problems for the baby are increased when, for some reason, there is difficulty in making a journey which can anyway be quite hostile. Although the baby books on the whole present a glossy picture of birth, the reality is sometimes different. Mothers these days are often not prepared for potential problems which may develop. Some people feel that expectant mothers are now told too much and that this may worry them, but there is indeed something to be said for an informed mother being an enabled mother. It must surely be a terrible shock when we are led to believe that having a baby is natural, and trouble-free, if this turns out not to be the case.

5 The loss of a Special Care baby

The trauma of seeing their child fighting for life is one that every parent hopes to avoid. The 'special babies' – those who begin their life under the intensive scrutiny of a Special Care Baby Unit (SCBU) are benefiting from the best medical, high-tech conditions possible, and yet some are just too ill to survive. The accounts detailed in this chapter describe many instances of doctors giving parents the opportunity to remove medical intervention and allow their babies to die in peace, in the certain knowledge that these little bodies cannot maintain their own lives.

BLISSLINK/NIPPERS, the bereavement group offering support for parents of Special Care babies, calculates that approximately 10 per cent of all children born in hospital are transferred to such units. This clearly includes many babies who need intensive nursing only for a very short time before being released into general care. It can certainly be a very lonely and distressing time, helplessly attending a child in Special Care while all other parents seem to be noisily celebrating the birth of their healthy babies.

About 1.5 per cent of the 700,000 babies born in the UK every year require the skills and equipment of an intensive care nursery in order to help them survive. For an average-size teaching maternity hospital, delivering about 4,000 babies each year, this means about two new babies each week. Many small pre-term babies (those born before 36 weeks gestation) survive with relatively simple treatment, but some need intensive care. Some 80 per cent of babies born before 30 weeks develop respiratory distress syndrome and require a ventilator to help them breathe. Thanks to this intensive care, the survival rate for even the smallest babies (less than 1kg, or 35.2oz) has improved, and for those above this weight the chances are even better.

The average stay for a baby in a Special Care Baby Unit is three weeks. Babies born as prematurely as $22\frac{1}{2}$ weeks have survived.

A basic crib costs in the region of £10,000, and five nurses are needed to run an intensive care cot around the clock. Every Special Care Unit in the country is short of equipment and often even more in need of nurses, so that expensive cots frequently have to stand empty. With so many items of specialised and costly equipment required by the neonatal intensive care unit, it is fortunate that charitable organisations exist. Prominent among them is BLISS (Baby Life Support Systems), which has a longstanding relationship with neonatal units and understands their needs.

More details of the services of the Special Care Baby Unit are outlined in *Born Too Soon*, a report produced by the Office of Health Economics, funded by the Association of the British Pharmaceutical Industry (see Bibliography). This report attracted widespread media coverage as it discussed many issues involved in the care of pre-term babies, including ethics and economics – basically the costs of saving the lives of very small and immature babies who could grow up to be severely handicapped. In response, BLISSLINK/NIPPERS produced a special report in February 1993, containing the opinions of contributors (parents, doctors and nurses) who had been involved with Special Care babies who later grew into healthy children.

Sandra, who leads us into this chapter, writes very bravely of the five months during which her daughter fought for life. The daily pain and worry are not mentioned, but can be read between the lines. Sandra does make the valuable point, however, that 'at least I have some wonderful ... memories that nobody can take away.' There is certainly an argument that every day of a child's life is a precious gift, and that to have a child even for a short time is a beautiful thing. The counter-argument, of course, is that the pain may be greater than ever when the end finally comes – that the temporary hopes raised may be cruelly shattered. But it is evident that Sandra would not wish to have missed out on Alison's short life; indeed all of our writers have been touched by the miracle of their babies, however briefly they survived.

Sandra

After having problems with my pregnancy from twelve weeks, with bleeding and not knowing what was causing it, I went to the doctor for an antenatal appointment on New Year's Eve. I told him of the pain I had had the night before; I said that it felt like the baby was trying to push its way out through my stomach. He told me I had to go to hospital right away and stay there until I had the baby. I thought I was in for a long wait as I was only 24 weeks pregnant.

When I got to hospital I was put on a drip and thought I would get some sleep. But the pain came back and it was getting stronger by the minute. I was taken to theatre for an emergency Caesarean section.

Alison Mary was delivered on New Year's Day at 3.35am, weighing 21oz (0.59kg), and she was fine. Next came the crunch, with the rush to find a cot for her.

They found a cot in Kent, so they called in the RAF to airlift Alison there. I first saw her when she was three days old, when I was transferred to Kent to be with her. Alison was given a 5 per cent chance of survival, but she had survived and was still fighting.

When she was five days old I went home as my other daughter needed me and I knew Alison was in good hands. I phoned the hospital every day and got to know the staff very well.

Alison was a week old when I had my first cuddle with her. At last she felt like my baby. I was also able to change her nappy, which was not as easy as I thought it would be as there were wires everywhere.

On 7 March Alison came off the ventilator and weighed 3lb 8oz (1.59kg). It was hard to believe. She stayed at Kent until 23 April, when they sent her home to our local hospital to get her off the oxygen and on to a bottle. It was the first time we could see the light at the end of the tunnel.

On 24 April Alison stopped breathing while I was visiting. This was the first time something had gone wrong, but she started breathing again in about two minutes. We knew her lungs were bad but this was the first time we had been given a name for the problem – BPD (broncho-pulmonary dysplasia). At the time we did not ask what this meant, but the next day we did and were told that we did not need to know, so I contacted NIPPERS and was sent a leaflet about the condition.

For the next five weeks things went from bad to worse. We got called in lots of times to be told there were only minutes until she died.

I asked to see Alison's consultant but he never turned up for the appointment. By now we had lost all our confidence and Alison was getting worse day by day.

On 19 May Alison was reventilated and sent to the children's hospital in Sussex. The staff there put us at ease and told us they were going to assess Alison for a fortnight. To start with things improved, but then got worse. She started to have fits whenever anybody touched her and her blood oxygen levels went dangerously low.

On Tuesday 4 June Alison weighed 7lb 7oz (3.07kg) and we were told there was nothing more that they could do for her. She had severe brain damage and her lungs had not improved at all. We switched the ventilator off and she died in my arms very peacefully.

But at least I have some wonderful photos and memories that nobody can take away.

Many of the babies in a Special Care Unit are there through prematurity. Kate's story is very different – she writes that 'the cruellest thing is that there was no clue ... I didn't know babies could be born and seem to be well ... and yet not be well at all'. Kate's daughter, Hannah, was born full-term but with a previously undiagnosed heart defect. This contributor speaks with great praise of the Special Care staff.

Kate

I gave birth to a supposedly healthy baby daughter on 23 February after a long and fairly difficult labour (no more difficult than a lot of other women's labours, though). I was full-term; in fact, our baby was late and I'd been induced, so she was a good weight at 7lb 4oz (3.3kg).

We called her Hannah Aimie. In retrospect, it was quite lucky it was a difficult birth as it meant we had a couple of hours after she was born, just the three of us, in the delivery room, while they waited to take the drips off me.

It had been a basically trouble-free pregnancy, although we had one major scare. When I had my routine 18 week scan the doctors thought there was something that might have indicated a chromosomal disorder, so I chose to have an amniocentesis, which turned out to be OK. However, I fell into the trap of thinking that this was a more or less sure-fire guarantee that everything was alright.

Anyway, we had a good first night. I fed Hannah and she seemed to be quite happy, albeit a bit bruised and bumped from the forceps. Thank goodness the policy in the hospital is to keep babies with their mothers. The next day was great too, although in the evening my husband Gerry was a bit concerned that she seemed to be panting a bit. I just put this down to it being so hot and stuffy in the ward.

That night was difficult. She wouldn't settle, but then none of the other babies did either. In the middle of the night the midwife took her to the nursery – she was obviously concerned but let me think that it was to give me a rest.

Hannah was brought back to me at 3.45am, when I gave her a feed (her last one as it turned out), and again she wouldn't settle so I took her into bed with me and we both fell asleep. In the morning a paediatrician came to see her and then we were just left. I was upset and worried as there was obviously something wrong.

Sister got her fed by a tube, as she couldn't suck, and got people up from the neonatal unit. Then they decided to take her down to the unit for tests. In a way I was relieved, but I was also very upset although I had no idea how serious it was. The sister was very caring and moved us into our own room, and she was also honest with us, telling us she was very worried – something we appreciated: it was better than being fobbed off.

Later the cardiologist broke the news that Hannah had a very rare, fatal heart defect and that there was nothing to be done. I remember thinking at the time how sensitive and caring he was. His manner and his way of talking to us were simply amazing. I remember just being flooded with disbelief, that someone would come running into the room saying they'd got it wrong. Then I remember thinking, 'I knew it, I knew it.' That was connected with the fact that I'd had an abortion 13 years ago when I was 17 and I'd always had the thought that if I had children there would be something wrong with them. But I also thought that I had to put all thoughts of myself and any repercussions to one side for Hannah's sake.

From then on, I can't praise the staff enough. The next thing was that we had Hannah baptised and confirmed in the neonatal unit. My dad collected Gerry's parents and, coincidentally, Gerry's best friend and his girlfriend arrived. It was the saddest christening imaginable. Then we had to decide to take Hannah off the ventilator. I want to stress how sensitive the staff were. We were left on our own in a quiet nursery-type room for as long as we wanted; they lent us a camera, which is something I wouldn't have thought of, and then we had a nice bedroom for the night. They also found somewhere for Gerry's parents to sleep. Anyway, no one knew how long Hannah would be with us, so we just wanted to make the time she had as easy for her as possible. Gerry, Hannah and I all slept together in this bedroom; Hannah was cuddled up on Gerry's chest. We all woke up the next morning. It was quite peculiar because one minute it was beautifully sunny and then the next it was snowing, almost as if specially for Hannah. We had all this day together and then most of the night. She died on her Dad's chest at about 10.30pm, three nights after she'd been born. I thank God that it was peaceful and that she had only been surrounded by love.

It is now 19 weeks since it happened and I do look back and wonder how we've got through it. She is always with us from the minute we wake up, and even when we're asleep. Gerry said something which I try to keep with me at all times: 'We must celebrate her, not mourn,' and it's true. She gave us so much joy and has completely changed our lives.

What I find particularly hard is going out and seeing pregnant women, babies, pushchairs, etc., and I feel so angry and hurt although I don't want anyone else's baby. The best thing for me has been reading – I read *When a Baby Dies* and its been my crutch. I joined SANDS immediately and the comfort of knowing there are people who know what you're going through and are just a phone call away is so important. Ultimately, the only thing that is going to help make it more bearable is time, although there are things that will help.

I just want now to have Hannah's brother or sister, not her back again, which is what I felt like in the first few weeks after her death, although of course I would do anything to have her back. Another awful feeling was isolation, which sounds quite common among bereaved parents. I felt so alone in my grief; that no one understood. That's why I think it is so important to contact a group.

For me, the cruellest thing is that there was no clue. I had heard of stillbirths and of babies being born poorly but I didn't know babies could be born and seem to be well – she looked so healthy, her bumps and bruises were clearing up well – and yet not be well at all. She was suffering from hypoplastic left heart syndrome. The other thing I have to say is that I felt completely abandoned by the professional services after I left the hospital. It really is a case of you have to know what you want and from whom and go after it – you can't wait for people to look after you.

Janet has sent two reports for us. The first details the life and sad death of her daughter, Emma.

Janet

The nightmare began on 17 December. I was 27 weeks into my second pregnancy. Two weeks earlier I'd had a routine scan (it was late because the hospital had lost the referral form) and been asked to return because they couldn't measure the baby's head properly as it was too low. It sounded so routine.

The scan was carried out by the senior radiographer and assistant, and they took lots of photographs. I still didn't realise anything was wrong, and couldn't understand why they kept asking if I was alright and when was my next antenatal appointment. It didn't occur to me to ask if the baby was OK, because I never thought they wouldn't tell me if it wasn't. All I asked was if the baby was the right size.

Shortly after I got home, my GP's receptionist phoned and said my doctor wanted to discuss my scan results with me. I assumed she meant the first scan, which had now been overtaken by the second one. As I look back now and write this, it seems incredible that I hadn't twigged something was wrong. But I still wasn't really worried; although I think I did have some idea things weren't totally OK, I thought the problems were with me, not the baby, and the worst thing to happen would be a few weeks in hospital.

After I was ushered into my GP's surgery, she sat down and told me gently that she was sorry but the scan showed that my baby was brain-damaged.

I was shocked and absolutely devastated, and burst into tears. My GP explained that I had developed polyhydramnios (too much amniotic fluid) because the baby wasn't swallowing properly. She offered me the choice of a termination, wait and see, or go to London for a more detailed scan.

She then arranged for my husband to be telephoned and handed me over to the midwife, who told me that the baby would probably be born prematurely because of the excess fluid which was making me so big.

The health visitor took me and my young son David home and left me to wait for my husband Clive to get back from work.

Fortunately, a friend called in and stayed with me until he came home.

We decided to go to London (about 150 miles away) for a further scan, and were assured by the community midwife that the doctor who would be doing the scan was the best in Europe at interpreting scan results, and that we should be guided by what he said.

On 22 December we drove to London. We were taken into the scanning room and about half a dozen students crowded round. Almost the first thing the doctor said was that the baby was not brain-damaged – what a relief. But there were other problems, and he thought it possible she had arthogryposis or a chromosome abnormality.

Ever since I was first pregnant we'd imagined having a little girl, and had called her Emma right from the start. The scan confirmed that she was a girl, and we were so pleased to be able to give her a name as we thought we might not have her for very long.

The doctor wanted to take a blood sample from the cord to test the chromosomes (amniocentesis would have taken too long) and at the same time to withdraw a lot of the excess fluid. Although taking off the fluid is risky and can set off labour, he said that without it I would probably go into labour very soon anyhow.

After the test had been done, the doctor asked us if we had a car with us and could we get to a different hospital in central London. When we asked why, we were told I was to have another scan at the special foetal heart-scanning unit. It wasn't until much later that I discovered that Emma's heartbeat had been very irregular; going first too fast and then too slow.

The doctor told us Emma probably had a condition which could prevent some of her muscles from working. If it only affected her arms and legs, it could be corrected with surgery; if it had reached her chest then she would die at birth. If the blood test results, due within a week, showed a chromosomal abnormality that was incompatible with life, he would recommend inducing labour as soon as possible. 'Is it possible that she will live for a while and then die?' I asked, as that seemed to be what I was most frightened of. 'No,' he replied.

At the second hospital we were told that there was nothing obviously wrong with the heart and we then drove home, getting back at about 10 o'clock at night.

We saw my GP on Christmas Eve and discussed the scan results with her. She made an appointment for me to see the consultant at the end of the first week in January; I wanted one sooner but because of the Christmas and New Year holiday nothing could be done.

Somehow we got through Christmas. By this stage I was enormous, exhausted, strained with worry and virtually unable to do anything. When the midwife came to see me the following week I said I wanted an earlier hospital appointment, but she couldn't do anything and said I would probably have the baby in a few weeks. I thought a few days was more likely.

On the morning of New Year's Day I started to bleed slightly. In many ways we were relieved; I could now go to hospital and be looked after properly.

At hospital I was told the cervix was still intact and that I was to be admitted for observation. Clive went home and I spent the afternoon on the antenatal ward. I was suffering from back pain which got worse and worse; the ward sister became concerned and sent for the doctor, who never came. Eventually, at about 6 o'clock, the midwife put me in a wheelchair and took me to the delivery suite herself.

The doctor examined me, confirmed I was in labour and went away again. When a midwife came to be with me, I asked if the doctor had told her how far on I was. 'Didn't she tell you?' she replied, 'You're about 6 centimetres.'

Labour consisted of an almost permanent but not too strong contraction. I was so stretched that the pain never went away, but gas and air took the edge off it until I made myself sick from having too much.

At one point the registrar came to see us and suggested that 'in view of the circumstances' we might wish to let nature take its course and not have a Caesarean if Emma began to get distressed during the labour. We didn't agree with this, and he then said that was the right decision.

By 10 o'clock I was 8 centimetres dilated and my waters still hadn't broken. The doctors decided that as she was so small I didn't need to be fully dilated and said my waters should be broken after the 10 o'clock shift change. The midwife who had been with us all evening went home (although I asked her to stay), saying, 'You could be another hour yet.'

As soon as the new midwife had taken over my waters were broken and I immediately began to push. Instantly, the room filled with doctors, nurses, incubators and all the paraphernalia that comes with a premature birth.

At 10.07 on New Year's Day Emma was born, at 29 weeks gestation. She weighed just over 3lb (1.4kg). The doctor took her straight away. I kept on saying, 'Is she alright?', but no one replied. As soon as she was on the ventilator and wrapped up for the trip to SCBU, they brought her over to me to see before they took her away.

I then had a retained placenta, not helped by the midwife whom I'd never got to know telling me to push and saying, 'You can't have a cup of tea until you've delivered this placenta.' But the cord was so thin it had snapped and my uterus was so stretched that there wasn't much chance, so I was given a general anaesthetic and taken to theatre.

When I came round I was taken up to SCBU on a trolley to see Emma, but I can't remember much. I was allowed to put my hands through the portholes and stroke her, and then taken to my room on the postnatal ward upstairs.

It was now about 2am. A nurse poked her head round the door: 'The newspaper wants the list of New Year's babies. You don't want her included, do you?' To my everlasting regret, groggy from the anaesthetic and emotionally worn out, I agreed with her and Emma was left out of the paper.

Memories of the next few days are dim. I spent most of the time in my room and very little on SCBU. I didn't know what to do when I got there and it didn't seem to make any difference to Emma whether I was sitting by the incubator or not.

The doctors were optimistic. They couldn't find anything seriously wrong with her. She was behaving as any other 29 week baby would. After a few days I went home and drove in to see Emma every day.

After just over a week she was off the ventilator, and on Sunday afternoon we had our first cuddle. We didn't have our camera with us, but another family did and took a picture of me with her. I missed the next couple of days because of a bad cold, and when I next came in she was back on the ventilator.

From then on she went slowly downhill. She began to have fits, but an EEG showed nothing. Her heartbeat was erratic, but the cardiologist could find nothing wrong. The ventricles in her brain had dilated and got worse, and we were told that she might be handicapped, although to what degree they couldn't say. She had more and more trouble breathing, and had to have her lungs suctioned out almost every hour. She was on drugs to sedate her, so she wouldn't fight the ventilation, and drugs to control the fits. But they could do nothing about the heart rate, as it alternated between going too fast and too slow.

When she was about four weeks old my husband and I should have visited together at the weekend, but David was ill with a tummy bug so I went on my own. When I arrived the doctor asked to see me. He told me that she wasn't getting any better, and that if she didn't show an improvement in the next few days we should consider withdrawing treatment. He then left me to drive the long journey home on my own.

When I got back I was in tears, and my husband and I accepted that we had reached the end of the road. We grieved for her that night as if she was already dead, and prepared to say goodbye. On Sunday morning we packed up the breast pump and went to the hospital, not knowing how long we would be there. When we arrived we were greeted with, 'She's much better,' and it was as if I had made it all up. No one realised the significance of the returned breast pump, that it meant we were giving up.

Emma held her own. The doctors were still convinced there was 'something' wrong with her, but didn't know what. They'd never seen a baby with her combination of symptoms, although they knew how to treat each individual problem.

She developed pneumonia, but recovered from it. I began to feel as if she would overcome anything.

On Valentine's Day, a Sunday, Clive and I went up together. It was a lovely sunny day and we brought a big box of chocolates for the nurses. Emma was doing very well. I sat and stoked her back and she stayed off the ventilator for about two hours. She was just over six weeks old.

The next day I stayed at home; I felt visiting every day was tiring me out too much and affecting David. Clive popped up to the hospital at lunchtime and came home in a bad mood. All evening he was depressed.

We were still awake, but in bed, when the telephone rang at 11.30. 'She's taken a turn for the worse; well, actually she's died.' We got dressed, wrapped David up in a duvet and took him to a friend, and drove to the hospital. When we arrived, the doors were locked and the porter wanted to know why we had come.

She was still in her incubator, which had been left on to keep her warm for us. We were taken to the 'quiet room' on the unit and she was brought in to us, dressed in a pretty white gown.

We both held her, kissed her and cried. A doctor and nurse were with us. The doctor was very offhand, as if this happened all the time. The nurse was more sympathetic, but we'd never met her before. We said goodbye to our little girl.

The next day we had to register her death, organise the funeral, see the head porter of the hospital, see the social worker, talk to the doctors again. I was very touched when my obstetrician came down to SCBU to see us and to offer a meeting with him whenever we wanted.

The social worker warned us that we would feel physically very tired, and she was right. The days seemed to pass in a daze, and nothing mattered.

We planned the funeral for the following Monday. The health visitor encouraged me to invite all my friends from the village; she said it would help them to express their feelings, and I'm glad I did. They didn't know Emma but they were there to support us. I'll never forget the sight of that tiny white coffin.

We had visited SCBU almost every day for six and a half weeks, and we always thought Emma was special to them too. But no one came to the funeral and no one sent a card or flowers. We had agreed to a post-mortem, and were told we'd be asked to come in and discuss the results in a few days. But nothing happened and they phoned on the morning of the funeral to say that they hadn't found anything and 'good luck this afternoon' (with the funeral).

After continual chasing from my GP we were given an appointment to discuss the post-mortem a few weeks later. The doctor said they could find no explanation for what had happened, and that it probably wouldn't happen again. At the same time, we brought along a donation to the unit from our friends and family (given instead of flowers). The senior nurse came to see us and said, 'I quite understand that you don't want to come on the unit.' We did, very much, but how could we say that after what she had said? We never did say goodbye to many of the nurses who had cared for Emma.

I'm writing this nearly six years after she died. I have come to terms with her death, but not with the care we were given during the pregnancy, while she was alive and after she died. I'm still very bitter about the way the scan results were communicated to us, the poor communication with the doctors while Emma was in SCBU and the lack of contact from the hospital after she died.

I've faced up to many of these problems. I complained to the Health Service Ombudsman about the scan, and received an apology from the hospital and a statement that I should not have been allowed to leave hospital after the scan without seeing a doctor. I even spoke to a consultant there about the communication problems, and have at least received an acceptance of what happened and an informal apology, but nothing really seems to clear the feelings of anger and hurt. I accept that Emma wasn't meant to live; but I cannot accept that the experience had to be quite as painful as it was.

Postscript: I got pregnant again soon after Emma died, but a blighted ovum was diagnosed at eight weeks and I was admitted to hospital for a termination. It took another seven months before I got pregnant again. After a very difficult pregnancy emotionally, Melanie-Ann Emma was born at term, followed two and a half years later by Matthew. Thankfully, we have three healthy children, but Emma is still an important part of our family.

In her second report, Janet goes on to analyse her relationship with the medical staff involved, particularly with SCBU. The experience is her own and happily not everyone is treated so badly, but it is important for us all to realise that any medical team is only as good as the individuals who make up that team. The doctors and nurses, no matter how strong their vocation, will inevitably have their own cares and concerns. It takes a very special person to be able to override their own problems in order to help others. Thankfully, most Special Care Units are made up of just such special people.

I find it hard to describe my relationship with the Special Care Baby Unit which cared for my daughter. In retrospect I consider the time she spent there to be uncomfortable and unhappy, yet I wish to remain involved with it.

After Emma's birth I found it hard to build up a relationship with the SCBU staff. The doctor who had been present at delivery did talk to me regularly for the first two weeks, but then suddenly disappeared for a fortnight. The nurses in the intensive care ward changed continually, and I hardly knew their names.

Many did not wear badges, or introduce themselves, and I wondered if they even knew which mum belonged to which baby. I desperately wanted to get to know them better: I wanted to feel more comfortable when visiting Emma, and I wanted them to like me so that they would look after my baby properly.

I tried to be present for ward rounds, but found that the doctors did not often acknowledge my presence. No one doctor seemed to be in charge of communicating with us, and at times it was hard to find anyone to talk to. My husband felt that if he walked into the ward and no one wanted to look at him, then Emma must be worse and there would be red ink all over her chart. There were inconsistencies in the attitudes of the doctors: some would make things look as black as possible; others tried to look on the bright side. I don't think anyone knew what was wrong with her, or if she would live, but there were many upsetting times and discussions that could have been handled more sensitively.

I was beginning to spend longer periods at the hospital; I would time my visits to coincide with nappy changes and other care, and was occasionally allowed to cuddle my daughter, if the nurse on duty was willing to take the trouble and could spare the time to supervise these cuddles. I never asked for a cuddle; I felt this treat had to be offered. But again, when I did hold her I didn't know what to do; it was not a relaxing contact, but watched and unnatural, accompanied by wires and tubes and monitors. At least I was beginning to spend more time touching her; holding her tiny hand and patting her back, and I now realise that she did respond to this, as she had fewer 'blue spells' when I was there.

I began to get to know some of the junior doctors and was feeling more comfortable with them, if not with the nurses, when three of the four senior house officers changed and it was back to square one; again, we were not introduced to the new doctors.

I was always asked to leave the ward when any procedure, even a blood test, was carried out, and it was a long time before I had the confidence to insist on staying; some procedures may have been upsetting, but so was waiting in the quiet room and imagining. I feel now that she should have had her mother there when all those needles were being stuck into her.

I do stay in touch with SCBU; I am a member of the parents' association and help with fundraising and coffee evenings, but I do feel out of place because the other active members have babies who survived. I desperately want something positive to come out of Emma's life and to be in an environment where I can talk about her without making people feel uncomfortable.

I have since met a new paediatrician at the unit, a meeting arranged by the obstetrician looking after me in a subsequent pregnancy when he realised how unsettled I still was about my pregnancy with Emma and the handling of her life and death. The new doctor was very patient and understanding, and went through her notes with us in great detail. He felt there had been something wrong with the 'wiring' of her heart; a freak abnormality whose cause could not be explained but that was unlikely to happen again. Since this meeting I have felt a lot happier about SCBU, that I have a better understanding of what went wrong and that other parents are being treated more sensitively than we were at times.

Vicki writes of her desperately sad experiences during the premature births of her two sons. The first was stillborn and the second lived for only a very short time. It is significant of many parents' attitudes that she writes that one day she may perhaps come to see incubators 'as life-savers rather than torture chambers'. Every parent of a 'Special Baby' questions the kindness and necessity of the intrusive medical treatment – to see a tiny, fragile baby being intubated or injected is heartbreaking, even though common sense tells us that it is imperative.

Vicki

Joshua was born on 18 March 1990. He was a much-loved and wanted boy; his arrival eagerly awaited by my husband Calum, myself and both sets of grandparents. He was born 16 weeks early, perfectly formed but dead. The doctors could offer no explanation. The shock of it all devastated me.

Joshua was cremated and his ashes scattered among the roots of an oak tree planted in his memory at a beautiful spot overlooking the River Dart.

Less than three months after Joshua's death I became pregnant again. The pregnancy had a tremendously healing effect on me. It was a very healthy pregnancy and I chose to believe all my friends' and relatives' encouraging words: 'You'll be alright this time,' they said, but at 24 weeks I began to feel less confident and asked my GP to check the baby's heartbeat. It was fine and I was told my nervousness was understandable as I had lost Joshua at 24 weeks. However, hearing the baby's heartbeat had failed to reassure me as much as I had hoped it would and a small loss of blood at 25 weeks made me worry.

On the first day of my twenty-sixth week I went to work as normal, although I felt rather low on energy. By the time I got home I was feeling very tired and, as Calum had gone away, I went straight to bed. A few hours later I woke up with a tummy ache. By 1am the pain was very strong and seemed to come in waves. I decided it would be a good opportunity to practise the breathing techniques I had learnt at last week's NCT [National Childbirth Trust] classes – not that these were contractions of course!

By 2am the pains were getting even worse and I phoned for my GP to visit. He realised immediately that I was well in labour. While waiting for the ambulance I phoned around to leave a message telling Calum I'd gone to hospital and then calmly packed a bag. That strange sense of calm that refuses to believe what is really happening is most extraordinary.

The ambulance rushed me to hospital. Within minutes of clambering on to the hospital bed my waters broke. Panic stations! Where was the doctor? Where was the special prem-baby equipment? As everyone dashed around me I could resist the urge to push no longer and at 3.51am on 25 November 1990 Jamie slithered into the world with a little cry. He was quickly wrapped, his cheek offered to me to kiss, then whisked away into the depths of the hospital. I lay on the bed in a stunned silence.

Minutes later Calum breathlessly rushed into the room expecting to see a second Joshua lying lifeless in my arms. He was overjoyed to learn that Jamie was alive and dashed off to see him. Soon afterwards I joined Calum in the room where our tiny frail son with paper-thin, transparent skin was lying on a rough-looking towel and being none too gently connected to tubes and needles. It was horrifying. I could hardly bear to look and had to prevent myself snatching him away from all the people in white coats who were obviously causing him so much distress.

Jamie had to be transferred to the Special Care Baby Unit at Exeter. His travelling incubator was wheeled into our room and a tiny hand reached out as if to wave. It was heartbreaking. I felt he was waving goodbye.

Some hours later I too was transferred to Exeter and found Jamie's tiny body still alive in the centre of a maze of medical equipment beeping, wheezing and pinging every few minutes. The noisy, harsh plastic and metal machines seemed such a crude imitation of the gentle soft womb Jamie had been safely enveloped within until so recently.

We were told Jamie was a fighter and although he was 14 weeks early and weighed less than 2lbs (0.9kg) he still had a 50/50 chance, and there was hope.

I just couldn't believe them. From the moment I'd looked down and seen his tiny newborn body between my legs I knew he was going to die. Calum, on the other hand, clung on to the slither of hope we'd been given. He proudly introduced Jamie to his parents and sister when they visited and sat next to his incubator all through that first night, willing him to live.

Next morning Jamie was still fighting, but we'd been told the first 72 hours were the most critical. By that afternoon, just 36 hours after his birth, Jamie was struggling and the oxygen pressure had to be increased significantly. When we tried to visit him with his grandparents, who had just dashed down the motorway from Kent, we were turned away and told we might be distressed by what we saw.

Shortly afterwards the paediatrician came to tell us Jamie had died – the oxygen pressure had been too great, his left lung had burst and his heart had stopped.

Jamie was brought in to us in a little Moses basket. He was dressed in the tiniest white babygro – still far too big for him. He looked beautiful and, for the first time, peaceful. Strangely, my predominant emotion at that time was one of relief. Relief that he was free from all the harsh machines that seemed to make him suffer so much.

Some days later Jamie was cremated in a tiny white coffin just as, only eight months earlier, Joshua had been. Jamie's ashes were scattered on the roots of a second oak tree planted close to his brother's.

I fell into a deep, sorrowful depression that lasted a year. My husband, family and friends were wonderfully supportive but no one except me could reach the wound that hurt so much.

An all-time low came in March 1991 when a hystero-salpinogram showed my uterus to be 'unicornate' and the most probable cause of my two babies' early deaths. (A unicornate uterus occurs when one half of the uterus has failed to develop, leaving a much smaller, tube-like space in which the baby has to grow. Lack of space forces the baby out, often months before its expected date.)

I found it so hard to contemplate conceiving a third child knowing that it would almost definitely have to spend considerable time in an incubator. Even if the child did survive, the chance of both physical and mental handicap would be considerable. Was it fair to impose these risks on the child?

I looked into the adoption process both abroad and within this country. I looked into the possibility of surrogacy and had sincere offers from a sister and a friend. But deep down I knew I had to have one last try myself. I hadn't known what was wrong with me during my last pregnancies. Next time I might be able to receive help that would give the baby a much greater chance of healthy survival than Jamie ever had.

It was a full twelve months after Jamie's death before Calum and I began to feel we could face the possible risks of a third pregnancy.

We are currently trying for a baby and I feel quite strong in my decision to do so, although I'm not free from doubts. Perhaps next time I will have a chance to come to terms with the way incubators are and will begin to see them as life-savers rather than torture chambers.

I still grieve deeply for the two lost little boys but I am beginning to see that the whole experience of their births and deaths was also an enriching one. I am able to smile again and enjoy the beauty of spring.

The excellent news is that Vicki later had a healthy daughter, Jemima, born at 35 weeks, who went home after twelve days in SCBU.

We close this chapter with words from Carolyn. Enormous strength seeps from her writing – we can add nothing, except to say that we feel honoured to have been touched by the warmth of it.

Carolyn
May–June 1991. I was 26 weeks into my first pregnancy and feeling wonderful when I woke up early one morning to find that I had been bleeding slightly. With the wisdom of hindsight I now know that this was a 'show'; at the time, though, I had not been to antenatal classes and, although extremely well

informed on the stage of pregnancy I was at, I had read no further in the books. I visited the doctor and after an examination he told me to go home and rest and call him later if anything changed. I felt confident it was just a minor hiccup, nothing that a day lying flat in front of the TV wouldn't cure. If only I'd known. By 11pm I was firmly installed in the hospital delivery suite in the full throes of labour. Of course the little tinker didn't arrive for some time. The doctors gave me drugs to stop me delivering so prematurely, steroids to strengthen him (specifically his lungs) in case he should arrive early and painkilling drugs for the contractions – but this baby was clearly on his way.

I spent the next week in hospital. For a while things would quieten down and then without warning labour would appear to start again in a serious way. At one point I even had an epidural administered, since we were all sure birth was imminent. On the sixth day things looked really stable. I'd had no contractions for 36 hours. The hospital had decided on a policy of non-intervention since I had grown intolerant to the drug that should stop labour and I was still only very slightly dilated, the same as when I had arrived a week before. I begged them to let me go home and swore I'd lie horizontal and do nothing for the next three months.

Gareth, my husband, came to collect me and as soon as I was installed (horizontal) on the settee he rushed out to buy a portable phone so that in the event of any surprises I could ring him from anywhere in the house. I say again – if only I'd known.

The moment I heard the car pull out of the drive I was off again. Oh, the pain. I squatted, I knelt, I lay on my back with all fours in the air. Then I needed the loo – boy, did I need the loo. I lumbered upstairs between contractions (how could I know about bearing down? – I never got to the classes). Fortunately, and I thank God, he wasn't quite ready to arrive. I just had time to call a taxi, scream all the way to the hospital, and within 20 minutes had delivered the most beautiful dark-haired, olive-skinned little boy named Aaron Lloyd.

That was only the beginning. How can I begin to tell you about the next six days? That beautiful little bundle of love had fought so hard to get out into the world, but he just wasn't quite cooked – didn't he know when he was on to a good thing? He should have stayed put. Naturally he was instantly taken off to the Special Care Unit to the loving and capable hands of a huge team of paediatricians and dedicated nursing staff. We weren't able to see him for four hours and before we did the senior paediatrician came to see us and warned us that the chances of his survival were 60/40 against, that although he looked so beautiful and his 2.5lb (1.14kg) was a good weight he still had a long, long way to go. Didn't he just. He lay so tiny, so helpless amidst a mass of wires, tubes, bleepers, monitors ... a machine to breathe for him, a machine to measure this and another to stabilise that. I couldn't look, I just couldn't bear it. I just ran, to gather thoughts, strength, courage. But the love, oh the love! I never knew I could feel so much love, almost too much, it spilled out of every part of me. I couldn't stop it or contain it – completely beyond my control. I had to learn that love so deep brings pain even deeper, so intense that it physically hurts.

And so began a long haul, a knife-edge walk. We watched, adored and prayed for this little being with every breath in us. He was so strong, so lively (when he was not doped to the full) and, my God, so beautiful. We adjusted ourselves to the months that would follow, the months of to-ing and fro-ing to the hospital, spending every waking moment with Aaron. We looked forward to Christmas, to his crawling, walking, talking. To his games, his education, his girlfriends. It felt so good.

He had good days and bad days, peaceful nights and terrible nights. One particular night he was so bad that we thought he'd certainly not make it through till morning, but he did. What a fighter. By 7am he had settled down again and everything looked so much more hopeful. I pottered home feeling more positive and hopeful than I had for a week.

As I drove back to the hospital at lunchtime I reflected that this was how it was going to be from now on – I would know every bump in the road en route to hospital before these long months were over. Gareth was already there at the reception of the Special Care Unit. If I hadn't been walking on clouds, so full of hope, I would have registered the sheer panic on his face, the utter relief when he saw me. He took me by the arm. 'He's having a really tough time in there, Carolyn, they're operating, they're doing everything they can.' And so we went into the waiting room. It hadn't sunk in. Aaron had already been through two blood transfusions, two lung puncture operations and if he could get through last night – well, he could get through this. Eventually the door quietly opened and in came

the ward sister and a female doctor with whom, until now, we had had very little contact. The doctor sat down gently on a coffee table facing us and looked intently into our eyes.
God, this was it and I wasn't ready to hear it.

'Well, we really have done all we can for Aaron and this is it now; there is nowhere left for him to go. He has fought so hard, but we've lost the battle. I think the best course of action now is for you to spend some time with him, you can pick him up and cuddle him now if you like. Then, when you are ready, when you say so, we will turn off the ventilator and let him go with some dignity.' They left us then. We held each other so tight. There were no words we could say. Moments like that are beyond words.

We moved silently into the hot-room where Aaron was and the nurses put screens up around his little cot so that we could have some privacy. As I looked into their faces I saw hurt there too. God, what a job they have. As the afternoon went on I think buckets of tears were cried by everyone, except Gareth and I. Somehow it was too public and we weren't ready. The sister picked Aaron up and wrapped him in a blanket and handed him to me. He was so light, so fragile, but he looked so content. We both held him for a bit but it felt awkward, he was still all wired up and we had to sit virtually in the incubator in order not to stretch any of the wires, drips etc. ...

I cannot remember the exact sequence of events. I know that my dad arrived, then my mum and later Gareth's mum too; and I know that it wasn't long after first holding him that we asked them to turn the ventilator off. Four overriding memories of that afternoon remain that I would like to share.

First was the overwhelming feeling as I held Aaron and kissed his face, his hands, his head, that if I could just take him home with me I could love him better. I would hold him so tight and give him so much, I really felt that I could love him back to life.

Second was the strength of that love, so much love that I wished I could die in order to give Aaron the chance of life. I never believed anyone could really feel that, but now I know that they can.

Third, my need for Gareth. At one point, he left the room; it was stifling in there and he needed some space. He was gone for a matter of moments, but if felt like forever. I have never felt so lost and completely alone as I did in that time without him.

Finally, the physical pain I felt as Aaron died. Half of me felt so relieved: relieved that his life was over, that he'd been released to a better kind of life. The other half hurt so deeply that I cannot describe it. In those hours and days that followed his death I thought I would never ever feel better.

September 1991. The summer that has just passed simply smothered our lives with a blanket of grief. We just got on with our lives – getting up and going to work took every ounce of spare energy that we had. Now I know how exhausting grief can be. We reached a point where we just kept ourselves precisely to ourselves, we didn't want to see anyone, to have to talk, to have to think, to have to go over everything again in order to salve other people's concern. It was too exhausting.

During those summer months after Aaron's death there were things that I found really helpful and things that really enraged me. I suppose that is why people always find it so hard to 'find just the right thing to say'; because 'the right words' change from hour to hour and minute to minute. What you think will help, I may not be ready to hear. What warmed me were the cards and letters where people simply wrote what they felt – no frills, nothing fancy. It made us appreciate what really good and loving friends we had. It felt good when people would just come up and say, 'I just wanted you to know how sorry I am and how hard I have been thinking of you.' They didn't want me to talk back, to explain, even to thank them – they just wanted to offer their support.

What did I find hard? People who couldn't look me in the eye and I therefore had to go out of my way to accommodate and reassure them in order for us to be able to resume a normal relationship. Those who told me that 'these things happen for a reason and if I can't see it now then I will in years to come'. I know these folks are well-meaning and, believe me, I am the eternal optimist and I *can* find *some* good out of all this tragedy but, tell me, what possible true reason or consolation can there be in such a tiny, beautiful, innocent little boy being plunged half-cooked into the world and then plucked away so rapidly? It's a bloody awful thing to happen, to him, to us and everyone concerned. It should never have happened and I will never see a reason for it, ever.

The final thing that made me bite my tongue and want to run screaming away was when a well-intentioned relative said, 'I do know what you're feeling.' 'You don't! How can you? You haven't asked me how I feel, I haven't told you and I'm not quite sure myself how I feel, so don't presume or even try to imagine you know what I'm feeling. How can you *possibly* know my pain?'

Still, all that is past now and life, as they say, goes on. There is not a day goes by when I don't think of Aaron. He is part of our family, he will never be forgotten and he can never be replaced. But that dull ache is fading and mostly I am left with a warm glow of love and acceptance. I still cry, of course I do, but it isn't the painful desperate crying of a few months ago but more often than not just a wave of love and sadness at that beautiful child we have lost.

After Aaron died he was sent to Oxford for a post-mortem. We felt a wave of relief when the results came back showing that he had been perfect in every way, it was just that his lungs weren't developed enough to cope out in the big wide world. The cause of his death was stated simply as 'extreme prematurity'. When he was cremated we placed a wreath on his tiny white coffin. It was made with blue and white flowers in the shape of a cross and on the card we wrote: 'Aaron, during your brief stay with us you brought so much love, joy and happiness. We will never forget. Be happy. Mummy and Daddy.'

June 1992. It is nearly a year to the day since Aaron died. Most of the year I have spent giving life to this tiny four-week bundle in my arms. Bryony Elizabeth we have called her, and of course she is absolutely beautiful. How quickly I have taken her existence for granted, how quickly I have forgotten all those weeks in hospital when I struggled to get her to stay put for just a little longer. I counted every extra day of pregnancy as a blessing and lived in the absolute fear that Bryony would be another 'Special Care' baby – I didn't want her ever to have to go near an incubator. I prayed to God that she would be born in my arms and stay in my arms – my prayers were answered.

Someone once said to me that a child is not ours to own, he is not a possession. A child is simply lent to us by God. That is one of the most beautiful and comforting thoughts that I keep in my mind when I think of Aaron and, I hope, that I shall be able to hold on to as Bryony, God willing, grows up with us.

6 Announcements and funerals

Announcements

Alongside the many emotional traumas faced by parents following a stillbirth or neonatal death, there are also practical issues to be faced. One of the difficulties met by parents who have experienced the birth of a very ill baby, or a stillbirth, is how to tell people. The shops are full of beautiful birth announcement cards which are all designed for celebrating the arrival of a child, but often these seem inappropriate if the baby's life is complicated by disability and illness, or if he or she dies while still in the womb or at birth. But the parents have had a baby, whether it is alive or dead. Relatives and friends often do not know how to respond to the news: they may (with the best of intentions) fear that if they acknowledge and celebrate the birth, it will further upset the parents, but not to acknowledge it will offend even further.

From the reports gathered in this book, it is clear that parents want to be acknowledged as just that – new parents – and that it is dreadfully hurtful for people to avoid the subject, or to pretend that the event never happened. The overwhelming feeling which comes across from the reports we received is that parents see the birth of their child as a supremely important event. This is the case whatever the outcome. After all, the parents have been expecting the baby for nine months or more, and the mother will have felt her baby moving and growing inside her. The baby is a real person. All births are to be celebrated; the death of a baby is devastating, but needs to be marked as the loss of any other person would be.

Sue and Chris, whose story of the birth and death of their daughter, Rachel Alexandra, is recounted in chapter 3, have kindly agreed to us reproducing their homemade birth and death announcements which were created by Chris on his word processor. Not everyone will have access to such a machine, but a handwritten message, photocopied, may be an alternative. We use them here to provide examples for parents of a very sick baby who may not know quite what to say to people around them but want to prepare them for the worst, or for those who wish to announce a stillbirth. By announcing the birth, Chris and Sue were inviting people to contact them with their congratulations on the arrival of Rachel. However, by including with the announcement a letter detailing Rachel's condition, they were also letting people know that they needed support and giving them some idea of what sort of card or message to send. This, in turn, made hurtful comments, or the danger of people ignoring the birth for fear of offending, much less likely.

Sue and Chris
are surprised to announce the birth of their daughter
Rachel Alexandra
at
8.51 pm on Friday 25 June 1993
10 weeks ahead of schedule and weighing 1lb and 10oz

The letter accompanying the death announcement was kept fairly brief and factual. It informed people of the events in Rachel's short life, announced that her parents were taking a holiday and needed some time to themselves, and included an acknowledgement to the hospital where Rachel was born and cared for. Sue and Chris also asked for donations for the Special Care Baby Unit: a particularly thoughtful touch, as such units rely heavily on public donations for their unstinting work. This also meant that people felt not quite so helpless, in that they could do something positive to celebrate Rachel's life.

Sue and Chris
regret to announce the death
of their daughter
Rachel Alexandra
25th June – 2nd August 1993

Sue and Chris were perhaps more thoughtful than many people feel they would be in such a situation. If the parents feel unable to create such announcements, then a close friend or relative may feel that s/he can assist in a practical way with this. On the reverse of the announcements, following Sue and Chris's lead, details of the baby's condition and treatment so far could be given, to answer any questions that relatives and friends may have.

Funerals

One of the many regrets of parents who lost their babies many years ago is that they were not given the chance to have a proper funeral, or to take part in the final ritual of saying goodbye. Thankfully, this has now changed. The arrangements for a funeral are often left to the father, particularly if the mother has had an instrumental or Caesarean delivery and is not feeling physically very well.

Our thanks once again go to Sue and Chris, who were keen to help other parents by sharing details of the service they used for their daughter, Rachel. The funeral service is an area which may be difficult for people to plan, particularly if they have no religious convictions. Parents will want to feel that they had an appropriate service and it is obviously an area which needs sensitive handling. A hospital chaplain or social worker should be able to assist, and may know of funeral directors who are particularly helpful in such situations. It is important for the service to be meaningful to the parents, because it will form a major part of their memories. Although Sue and Chris do not have a specific set of religious beliefs, they found the ritual and symbolism useful in helping them to deal with their grief and to do tangible things by which to remember their daughter.

Their particular service was a mixture of Christian and lay. Two lay readings from works by Morris West and Kahlil Gibran had particular meaning for the parents. Obviously, other parents may have special texts or songs which are deeply meaningful to them. By informing people beforehand of Rachel's birth and disability, Sue and Chris did their best to help people to understand the situation the three of them had faced. They were able to use a wonderful memento to their daughter on the front of the order of service, Rachel's handprint. This in itself poignantly illustrates Rachel's plight, from the smallness of her hand, to the angle of fingers one and four and the lines of her palm.

We hope that the thoughts shared by Sue and Chris assist other parents. They commented that the funeral was a 'joyous event', and made the point that some of the floral tributes were taken home and enjoyed. In this instance the couple then escaped on a quiet holiday, which gave them time to be alone with their thoughts and meant not having to contend with work, the people around them and everyday life. If other parents can afford it and find the idea useful, a holiday to start the process of recuperation is certainly a thought.

Martin and Vivienne, mentioned in chapter 2, also told us a little about the funeral of their daughter, Kieran.

> A hospital bereavement counsellor came to see us, to talk through the options. We are not religious, so decided on a Church of England vicar and a cremation service. The vicar visited us twice. The cremation service went as well as it could.

There was only one incident, when the undertaker started to carry the tiny coffin which Martin had planned to carry. He explained:

> I wanted to hit the undertaker. I was the one to carry Kieran's coffin; but it was the longest walk I've ever done. We scattered Kieran's ashes on Ashworth moor, as we didn't want a grave which would bind us to one area.

Martin will go up to the moor, particularly after a bad day at work, to think and remember Kieran in the beauty of the hills.

7 The way forward

The grieving process

Psychologists accept that grieving is a long process and that individuals must pass through certain stages before they can come to terms with their loss. Grieving (with help) often takes a year or two to reach a state of resolution. Society has generally been rather intolerant of grief and the whole process surrounding it, perhaps because it is little understood – strange really, given that we all encounter the deaths of our loved ones at some point in our lives, so we should be able to empathise at least a little.

It is ironic that people expect a woman to take pre-conceptual care and to be responsible during the 40 weeks of pregnancy, but conversely expect her quickly to come to terms with any loss at the end of this waiting period. Many of our early reports concern women who had little help with their grieving, and were generally expected to behave as if nothing had happened or as if they had delivered a live baby. At least one of those is today undergoing therapy to help her to come to terms with her loss of many years ago.

The death of a baby is also the loss of hopes and expectations during the preparation of pregnancy, and it might be that no one can truly understand it unless it has happened to them. Mourning is learning to live without a loved one, but can be very difficult in the case of a stillbirth because, while there is a great sense of loss, parents haven't fully known what is lost. They have never known their baby as an independently live individual. It has been termed 'the loneliest loss', as only the pregnant mother has really had daily contact and interaction with her baby.

Usually, we expect to die before our children – this is the natural order, the scheme of things. The death of babies is no longer a familiar occurrence, and many people will have no experience of it. It is in some ways then perhaps unrealistic to expect others to be able to comfort the bereaved, especially as they may have difficulty in coping with their own emotions. This inability can manifest itself as indifference, which can make it harder for the parents to cope.

Even with technological changes, the dangers of stillbirth and neonatal death are still higher within the manual working classes than the more sedentary middle-class groups; likewise, new parents under the age of 20 are more likely to experience a stillbirth than their older counterparts are. There seem to be basic health education messages here, and social welfare implications which need addressing. The differences in access to satisfactory healthcare may be partly responsible for the problem. The groups at risk are also less likely to have access to counselling facilities if they do experience a loss.

While not meant to be a thorough investigation of the counselling of grief, it is possible to tie the process to three stages. The first is the initial reaction of shock, numbness, confusion and denial when the fact of death is first realised. There is an immediate sense of loss as people react to the catastrophe, unaware of their surroundings, unable to think coherently. To most people, losing a child of whatever age is the most devastating incident they can imagine – suddenly, for the expectant parents, their worst fears have come true. For many, it will be their first experience of any bereavement.

This is followed by intense sadness, lack of motivation and depression or anger which may be suppressed (for many years in some cases) or targeted at certain individuals who have played a role in the pregnancy and birth of the dead baby. The targets are often health professionals. This may be difficult for the professionals concerned, who will need to develop strategies for coping, but it is in many ways worse if the anger is directed within the family, such as towards the husband or wife. There may be regrets about things said or done, or left unsaid. Fathers in particular may feel embarrassment at suddenly feeling a loss of control, something they may not be accustomed to. The couple may feel drained and empty with little support to offer each other, each grieving in different ways and at varying rates. They need all their energy reserves for themselves. The mother may also be recovering from a difficult delivery and have to deal with physical problems which are hard enough for any new mother: stitches, the production of breast milk and hormonal adjustments as her body returns to its non-pregnant state. There may be other practicalities to deal with, such as siblings, informing family and friends and arranging a funeral, which may not give couples time to examine their emotions.

The third stage is that of acceptance and resolution, a stage that many must feel they will never reach. Coming to terms with one's own loss often leads to the ability or desire to help others, such as becoming involved in a support group. This happened to a number of our contributors. Different individuals vary in the time they take to grieve. This depends upon their own personalities, other events and responsibilities in their lives, and the degree of helpful support they are given, if they want it. Not all people request counselling and it is less likely to be successful if it is pushed on someone who does not really want it. Even when the loss is accepted, the sadness can be surprisingly overwhelming and recurrent, and the sense of loss often never fades completely. It is said that nothing ever prepares us for our first child; how much harder then to accept the death of a child whom we have created.

When grieving is unresolved, as in a number of cases mentioned here, the effects are likely to be long term; this is borne out by many of the reports from women whose only help came late and then generally from voluntary agencies. Women have been, and continue to be, failed by the medical profession and health/social care agencies, although provision varies greatly according to geography, means of access and, something more difficult to change, the personalities of the personnel involved.

One of the most hurtful approaches towards bereaved parents is to expect them to 'snap out of it' – they need people to be there, ready to listen, to talk, to share tears and even some laughter. Some parents need to talk, others need to internalise their feelings. Denial is not particularly helpful. Ours is not the only culture which attempts to deny the existence of the stillborn baby or neonatal death as a complete person. All cultures and individuals develop their own ways of dealing with the situation.

A painful and traumatic birth experience can, and sadly does, put many excellent parents off having more children. Even today, when pain relief is widely available, childbirth can be physically difficult and emotionally distressing. How much more distressing then to find that delivery is long and arduous, the paediatrician is on standby and there is no live baby as an end result. Decisions not to have more children were surprisingly common among those who contacted us – after one loss, couples were often unable to bear the further possibilities of grief and physical distress, and were anxious about the effects of this upon the marital relationship.

This is an area where many women later had regrets and where adequate counselling might have led to a life-changing decision. Conversely, other women felt they would only begin to heal when they had a healthy baby in their arms; here, appropriate medical advice, and in some circumstances genetic counselling, seems essential.

When should a couple try for another baby? Unless there are medical indications otherwise, as soon as possible is fine if that is what a couple want, and if they want the baby for itself, not as a replacement or substitute. The best time is perhaps when the death is accepted. Outside agents may pressurise a couple to 'try again', but their loss is very personal, it may have repercussions on their relationship (see below). Research at the Tavistock Institute has shown that parents rushing into a next pregnancy can suffer many problems. At three months the pain is likely to be very great; what parents actually want is the baby who died. They need time to grieve and think about that baby before thinking about another. Fortunately, one stillbirth or neonatal death does not automatically mean another, and many contributors have reported that they later went on to have a perfectly healthy pregnancy and birth with a resulting live baby. This does not replace the lost child, but offers hope for happiness in the future.

Organisations such as SANDS fulfil an excellent self-help function, as do most voluntary agencies in this field. SANDS has support groups in many areas and also offers individual support. It also, to its credit, raises funds to equip special rooms for bereaved parents in many areas. Perhaps what is needed is a group with the role of persuading health authorities to improve practices and procedures following stillbirth or neonatal death.

Losing a baby can have a shattering effect on a relationship. While many people believe that such a loss can strengthen the bond between a couple (and in some cases it does), the overwhelming experience seems to be that relationship problems either occur or deepen as grieving takes place. One problem is that women often try to protect men from knowing their pain, so that men can feel marginalised and shut out.

The great range of feelings aroused by the loss of a baby at the start of his or her life – from sadness, depression and guilt, to anger, revulsion at the thought of a death occurring within one's body (an aspect mentioned by a number of contributors), and fear of the inability to have live children – means there is a great deal for any couple to contend with. Single women may have particular problems of their own, and no immediate support from a partner. However, partnerships do not always provide the support network needed and can simply add to the difficulties.

While it is known that a stillbirth or neonatal death has a profound impact on a woman, it is difficult to assess exactly how it affects a man in a relationship. Sadly, there seems to be little research into this – which is not to say that men's reactions and feelings are not important, simply that there is no hard and fast information we can draw upon. But it does seem that the different experiences of men and women can often exacerbate relationship problems. Men differ considerably in their ability to empathise with their partners' emotions. Many do not feel a pregnancy is 'real' until the baby is born, and some not until he or she begins to be active and respond to them. It is the woman who has experienced the physical symptoms of pregnancy and has felt the baby alive within her, developing and growing. She may also have changed her lifestyle in certain ways, such as giving up drinking and smoking, or adopting a healthy diet to help sustain her baby; things which a father does not have to do in the same way, and which further foster a sense of attachment and closeness to the child.

The extent to which the woman shares her pregnancy and communicates what she is feeling may have some bearing on a couple's joint response to the loss of their baby. They may either pull very much together or instead find they are trying to cope with the turn of events quite separately, and in ways which the other partner may find excludes them and is hurtful. For example, one partner may wish to talk about the baby and display photographs; the other may not wish to have any reminders around the house.

There may be other underlying problems, all of which could be improved by a knowledge and understanding of the situation. For instance, the partners may have had different attitudes to the pregnancy; not all couples want family commitments to the same degree. Communication may be difficult – there can be people who have been married for many years who still do not communicate their problems to their partners. Family and other significant people may have an effect, and indeed the comments of parents and grandparents following a stillbirth or neonatal death can unwittingly be particularly hurtful and damaging. Social and financial circumstances may also have a bearing: a number of

women who responded to our request for information had decided
to be stay-at-home mothers, and then suddenly found themselves
with no baby and no outside employment – almost totally
redundant, feeling empty. Others who returned to work found it
difficult to accept that some colleagues could behave as if nothing
had happened. Finally, the roles each partner plays with respect
to the other may undergo dramatic change. For example, if a
woman has tended to be the strong one within a relationship, but
now suddenly needs strength from her partner, this may be
something of a reversal of the roles which usually work for
the couple.

Some of our contributors commented that their marriages had
not survived the devastation of losing a baby; others seemed to
find increased strength in their partnership following the trauma.
For some couples, outside help can work with them to maintain
a relationship. For example, Relate (formerly the Marriage
Guidance Council), while not specifically a service or charity for
bereaved parents, does have trained counsellors to help in every
aspect of relationship difficulty. Relate can work with couples
during the aftermath of the event over the long term, for weeks
or months, when the consequences unfold. This can be particularly
useful because this is often a time when support from family and
friends begins to dry up, with people assuming that the couple
should be taking steps to recover from their loss. This is not
usually meant to be unkind, but is frequently because others do
not know how to cope with continued grieving and do not realise
that the process can take a long time to resolve itself. It is in these
circumstances that outside support can be positively beneficial.

We are very grateful to Relate for the help given us in compiling
this book, particularly in the provision of anecdotal evidence
gleaned from the group's work with grieving couples. It should
be stressed that Relate regards client confidentiality as extremely
important and no specific case material has been disclosed by the
organisation.

Recommendations

Thankfully, many of the issues raised by our contributors are
now being addressed. Grief is a very painful experience and
unfortunately very common. Annually in the UK, around 620,000
babies are born alive, but one in every 100 dies before (after the

twenty-fourth week of gestation), at, or soon after birth – about 7,000 babies a year.

Back in the 1980s, a number of recommendations were made for the care of the mother following a stillbirth and many hospitals have worked quite hard to implement these. Generally, parents these days will know if their baby has died in the womb, so the grief and loss begin before birth. It is a lonely loss and emphasis tends to be woman-centred, as only the mother has experienced the baby at first hand for any length of time. This is also true to an extent in the case of a neonatal death in Special Care. When a baby has been rushed from the delivery room to the Special Care Unit, parents may feel that they have little chance to be physically close to him or her and essential equipment can become a barrier, especially if the mother is also recovering from an operative delivery and cannot move about freely. (This emphasis on the mother is not to underestimate the strength of emotion which involved fathers will have about their loss.)

The Kohner report made the following recommendations. Many have been implemented, but resources are of course ever limited, and the issue continues to be addressed by the Child Bereavement Trust in the 1990s.

1. Parents should have a choice of place to stay during their time in hospital. If they are on a labour ward, they may hear other babies cry and find this distressing, so they should be prepared for this. However, some people will prefer to be around babies as it makes their own experience meaningful – they did, after all, give birth to a baby. *Choice* is thus the operative word, although parents may be too stunned to make that choice at first.

2. Women in labour are offered painkilling analgesia. This is also the case where the baby has died in the womb, and parents need to be able to make an informed choice with assistance from staff – account should be taken of the physical and emotional pain. For some women, the pain of childbirth makes the event more real for them and gives them something to hold on to mentally or emotionally, a memory of their baby after the event. Others will not want any pain, and feel that if there is not to be a live child they should at least be spared physical pain.

3. For the delivery, two midwives should be present and they should undertake to make the birth experience as fulfilling as

possible. The management of the labour needs prior discussion with the mother, who may well have a birth plan.

4. After the birth, the baby should be tidied and presented. She/he should be handled gently, named and later placed in a cot. It is important for parents to see and hold their baby, and to be prepared for what they may expect in the case of any abnormality. They may need reassurance on this point, and the offer to see their baby should be made more than once. Among the contributors to this book, parents were often reluctant to see their babies, assuming something monstrous rather than, to all appearances, a normal baby. When parents did not see their babies there was often later regret; this did not seem to occur when parents came round to the idea of seeing their babies, and of course some wanted to do this straight away.

5. There should be family involvement, with the partner able to stay with the mother (and other family members too, if requested).

6. Sedation should only be given if wanted. For some parents, it will help; for others, it will delay the grieving process.

7. Mementoes, such as locks of hair, photographs and handprints, should be offered or kept in case notes, along with a blessing certificate or entry in the book of remembrance if the hospital arranges the funeral. It is often helpful to the family if midwives or staff attend the funeral, and for parents to know where their child is buried.

8. The mother should be given the choice of a single room or ward and she should have contact with staff, who need to make time to listen. A number of reports have suggested that mothers prefer privacy, with unrestricted visiting. A staff response offers proof that the baby was a person. It is good for staff to express their sorrow. Parents then feel that their baby's life had meaning to others too. Parents should be aware that they can see their baby at any time before the funeral. Some will want to see their baby many times; for others, once will be all they want and further visits may increase their distress, so all parents must be treated as individuals. Parental consent is needed for a post-mortem; this request should be made by a doctor who knows the people concerned rather than a stranger. The 1993 Yorkshire Television film *Empty Arms* provides an excellent example of good practice (see Bibliography).

For health professionals dealing with a baby's death, it should be noted that body language is important. Health carers can say as much by touch as by speech. It should also be remembered that a baby is a baby when the mother thinks of it as such, not according to medical definitions, and the use of terms such as 'spontaneous abortion' to explain a previous miscarriage may be devastating to the parents.

Many bereaved mothers have expressed the fact that they felt embarrassed, failures, as if they didn't belong. Social expectations for people to become parents are strong, and it is thought by many that becoming a parent should be a straightforward process. When all around you are having babies, it is easy to see why such feelings of failure may arise. Stillbirth is an individual and personal experience, and this is highlighted by the inability of many midwives and lay people to discuss and communicate on the issue.

For those parents who have encountered unhelpful attitudes, it is worth noting that there are a great number of caring health professionals out there. An excellent article by Sue Alexander which appeared back in 1987 (see Bibliography), makes the valid point that care-givers have their own grief to cope with too. The article, describing how one student midwife approached working with a bereaved family and dealt with her own grief and sorrow, is well worth a read.

For parents wanting to support themselves, the Child Bereavement Trust (see chapter 8) offers an excellent information pack, sensitively produced, suggesting ways in which you may want to remember your baby's life in a positive way that will assist in the long-term healing process and be a permanent reminder of the life you created, however short it was.

Preventing stillbirth and neonatal deaths

Is there any action which may be taken antenatally to improve the chances of a healthy baby? Antenatal care is now acknowledged to be better than ever before, with improved social conditions and education, supervision of 'at risk' mothers, screening, genetic counselling, early detection of many abnormalities, active management of difficult labours, monitoring and better staff training. But, as ever, there are groups of people who will not have access to all this. It is hard to know how to reach them.

Not all commentators agree that it is improved medical care which has made the experience of birth safer for the baby. Until about 1870, fertility was high and stillbirths and neonatal deaths were accepted as inevitable, sometimes even welcomed as a form of birth control. In difficult deliveries, doctors would often sacrifice the life of the foetus, if necessary, to save the mother. As birth rates began to decline, infant survival became more of an issue. However, some would suggest that changes in social conditions have had a far greater effect than medical advance.

Some experts believe it was the elimination of extreme poverty, together with increased nutrition and the better health of mothers, which cut the number of stillbirths and neonatal deaths. Increased rest also had an effect. There was, and still is, a close association between high obstetric mortality and lower social class, with poor nutrition the material causal factor. Risks of perinatal death from birth trauma, asphyxia and placental insufficiency increase with maternal age, especially in first pregnancies and in those lasting longer than 40 weeks – induction and the use of Caesarean deliveries may be useful in such cases.

It is important to try to ensure that all women take up the regular and high-quality antenatal care at their disposal under the National Health Service, and that appropriate diagnostic tests are offered to those known to be at risk. Antenatal care is recognised as one of the best forms of preventive medicine, and can offer the appropriate professional support to pregnant women and extra help where it is needed. This is true both within a hospital and out in the community.

GPs, midwives and hospital antenatal clinics can help to ensure a high level of take-up by sensible appointment systems and a patient-centred approach which encourages women to attend clinics. There is an increasing tendency towards shared care, with most appointments taking place at the local health centre rather than the hospital; and domino care, where a team of community midwives are responsible for the care of their patient. This informal system is more user-friendly and works well alongside the system of patient-held maternity records.

8 Where to get help

There are a number of organisations which provide much-needed support for bereaved parents. The list here is not comprehensive. There may, for example, be local support groups which are not included here, or counselling available through particular hospitals. Health visitors and libraries may be useful sources of information, while the care that GPs can give should not be underrated.

For parents

Association for Spina Bifida and Hydrocephalus (ASBAH)
ASBAH House, 42 Park Road, Peterborough PE1 2UQ
Tel: 01733 555955
ASBAH provides advisory and welfare services, practical assistance and information, and also maintains a team of trained fieldworkers to support new parents and individuals. It produces leaflets, booklets and newsletters.

BLISSLINK/NIPPERS Bereavement Group
17-21 Emerald Street, London WC1N 3QL
Tel: 0171 831 9393/8996
BLISSLINK/NIPPERS aims to offer support and information to parents of premature and sick newborns, and also to staff working with these babies and their parents. It can provide support, organise workshops and arrange memorial services at the request of parents.
    Its sister organisation is BLISS, which raises vital funds for the essential pieces of equipment needed by babies requiring complex intensive care.

British Association for Counselling
1 Regent Place, Rugby, Warwickshire CV21 2PJ
Tel: 01788 578328

If you feel you need counselling, then it is important to seek help from an approved counsellor in your locality; the Association can help with information on where to go.

British Humanist Association
47 Theobalds Road, London WC1X
Tel: 0171 430 0908
Can help with arrangements for non-religious funerals for neonatal deaths and stillbirths.

The Child Death Helpline
Tel: 0171 829 8685
This is for anyone affected by the death of a child and is based at the Great Ormond Street Hospital. It is staffed by bereaved parents. Open Monday and Thursday, 7pm–10pm.

The Compassionate Friends
53 North Street, Bristol BS3 1EN
Tel: 01179 539639 (helpline), or fax outside office hours 01272 665202
The Compassionate Friends is an international organisation of bereaved parents offering friendship and understanding, comfort and support to those who have lost a child or children.
  Befrienders will listen to the newly bereaved and offer a 'safe' situation where a wide range of emotions can be discussed; support is also offered through group meetings, one-to-one visiting and telephone or letter contact. There is also a quarterly newsletter, and help available for brothers, sisters and grandparents. There is no membership fee.

Cruse Bereavement Care
Cruse House, 126 Sheen Road, Richmond, Surrey TW9 1UR
Helpline: 0181 332 7227 (Monday to Friday 9.30am–5pm)
Cruse offers help and advice for bereaved people. Its concentration is not necessarily on losing a child, but the charity can help with the feelings of loss associated with all bereavement.

Maternity Alliance
15 Britannia Street, London WC1X 9JN
Tel: 0171 837 1265
Provides advice on maternity rights for women, including those who have had stillborn babies.
National Association of Bereavement Services

20 Norton Folgate, London El 6DB
Tel: 0171 247 1080
The Association produces a directory of bereavement services and can put parents in touch with an appropriate organisation when the choice seems bewildering.

National Association of Citizens' Advice Bureaux
115–123 Pentonville Road, London N1 9LZ
Tel: 0171 833 2181
Citizens' Advice Bureaux (CABs) offer free, impartial and confidential advice on any subject and may be your first port of call for advice and information if you feel that you have suffered negligence or poor treatment at your hospital. They hold details of local Community Health Councils and local solicitors specialising in medical negligence. Your local Bureau will be listed in the telephone directory.

National Childbirth Trust (NCT)
Alexandra House, Oldham Terrace, Acton, London W3 6NH
Tel: 0181 992 8637
The NCT offers postnatal support and may well have members in your locality who have been in a similar situation and can offer their support to you.

Relate
Herbert Gray College, Little Church Street, Rugby, Warwickshire CV21 3AP
Tel: 01788 573241, or see under Relate in your local telephone directory.
Relate offers confidential counselling for relationship problems of any kind, including those caused by grieving and bereavement.

Stillbirth and Neonatal Death Society (SANDS)
28 Portland Place, London W1N 4DE
Tel: 0171 436 5881
SANDS is a charity which provides support through self-help groups run by bereaved parents who work on a voluntary basis. They offer a telephone befriending service, regular group meetings in many areas and sometimes individual visits.

Local groups also carry out fundraising activities; for example, to equip parents' rooms in many hospitals so that bereaved parents may have some privacy in their grieving, and where both parents may stay together overnight while in hospital.

SANDS acts as a pressure group to bring to people's attention the plight of bereaved parents. For example, it was at the forefront in the fight to reduce the definition of stillbirth from 28 to 24 weeks. This was one area which parents felt strongly about – that a death at, say, 26 weeks might be treated as a miscarriage rather than a stillbirth. The charity also works with many health professionals to help them increase their awareness of the issues involved when a baby dies.

The SANDS telephone support service has someone to talk from 9am to 5.30pm and at other times the answerphone will give the names and telephone numbers of two people parents can ring. The organisation also publishes many books and pamphlets that may help bereaved parents and siblings.

Soft UK
48 Froggatts Ride, Walmley, Sutton Coldfield, West Midlands B76 8TQ
Tel: 0121 351 3122
Soft provides support, advice and information to families affected by Trisomy 18 (Edward's syndrome) and Trisomy 13 (Patau's syndrome). It also supports families with related disorders and chromosomal abnormalities, and has various publications. A bereavement support service is offered, as most babies with these conditions die shortly before or after birth, or during the first year of life, although there are exceptions.

Twins and Multiple Births Association (TAMBA)
PO Box 30, Little Sutton, South Wirral, West Midlands L66 1TH
Tel: 0151 348 0020
Tamba offers help and support to parents of twins, triplets, quads and so on. It has a good deal of experience of problems relating to twin and multiple births, where the risk of stillbirth or neonatal death is sadly greater than in single births. Publications are available and there are also local, regional and national meetings and study days.

For health professionals

Health professionals may be profoundly affected by the death of a baby before, at or shortly after birth. Sometimes they too will need support. (They are also, of course, free to contact other appropriate groups listed above for parents.)

The Child Bereavement Trust
1 Millside, Riversdale, Bourne End, Buckinghamshire SL8 5EB
Tel/Fax: 01628 488101
The Trust provides resources, information and training for health professionals. It was established in 1994 by Jenni Thomas, who has specialised in working with grieving families, counselling and nursing on children's wards, including Special Care. Something of a pioneer, Jenni has developed services in bereavement counselling to an excellent level. The aim of the Trust is to ensure all hospitals can offer counselling and staff training.

Counselling, Help and Advice Together (CHAT)
Royal College of Nursing, 20 Cavendish Square, London W1M 0AB
Tel: 0171 629 3870/409 3333
Offers a confidential counselling service for all nurses.

National Association for Staff Support
9 Caradon Close, Woking, Surrey GU21 3DU
Tel: 01483 771599
Offers support information for health service staff.

Neonatal Nurses Association
Room 7, A Block, Forest House, Berkeley Avenue, Nottingham NG3 5AF
Tel: 01159 602494

Royal College of Midwives Trust
15 Mansfield Street, London W1M 0BE
Tel: 0171 580 6523

Glossary

AFP test
The alphafetoprotein test is not always carried out routinely these days. AFP is the protein produced in the liver and gastro-intestinal tract of the foetus. It passes into the mother's bloodstream and may be measured by a maternal blood test between the fifteenth and twentieth weeks of pregnancy. A raised level suggests possible abnormalities such as spina bifida; a low level may be indicative of Down's syndrome.

Amniocentesis
The withdrawal of a small amount of the amniotic fluid surrounding the foetus in the womb, in order to test it for the presence of conditions such as Down's syndrome in the foetus.

Anti-D
This is an antiserum containing antibodies against Rhesus (Rh)D factor (which is present in the blood of those who are Rh positive). It is given to a woman who has Rh negative blood after she has given birth to a baby who is Rh positive (it may also be given to any pregnant woman who has had an amniocentesis, bleeding or miscarriage if there is a chance she has been exposed to foetal blood cells.) It means that the risk of the woman forming antibodies against Rh positive blood is lowered; if not checked this could affect a subsequent pregnancy.

Apgar Score
A scoring system used at birth to assess the wellbeing of the newborn baby. It takes into account breathing, colour and muscle tone. Most healthy babies score between 7 and 10. The score is reassessed five minutes after the birth.

Arthogryposis
A deformity caused by the shrinkage of tissue in skin, muscles and tendons, leading to damage and restriction of movements.

Breech position
A position adopted by a foetus in the womb whereby its head is at the top of the uterus instead of at the cervical entrance. This means that unless the foetus can be moved before birth, the baby's bottom will emerge first, rather than the head, and this can cause birth injuries.

Broncho-pulmonary dysplasia
Abnormality of growth of the bronchus, a large air passage in the lung starting at the end of the trachea (windpipe), which impedes the passage of air. The abnormality will vary in severity.

Counselling
While a number of people have counselling skills which may help parents, counselling should only be undertaken as professional intervention. Information is available from the British Association of Counselling.

D&C
A D&C is usually offered after a miscarriage, or for certain womb disorders. It is the scraping away of the endometrium (lining) of the womb, usually carried out under general anaesthetic.

Doppler scan
This special type of scan measures frequency changes and so, for example, can check the rate of blood flowing through a blood vessel, or the beating heart of a foetus in the womb.

Down's syndrome
A chromosomal abnormality which results in mental handicap and a characteristic physical appearance. It is caused by an extra chromosome 21 (i.e. there are three of these chromosomes instead of two). About one in 650 foetuses have Down's, but many mothers are screened for the condition during pregnancy.

Dysplasia
An abnormality of growth, which affects the size, shape and rate of growth of an organ. Broncho-pulmonary dysplasia, for example, means that the lungs don't develop as they should.

Eclampsia
A fairly rare, serious condition of late pregnancy, labour and delivery, this is a complication of the less severe pre-eclampsia (see separate entry) and is believed to be caused by excess fluid swelling in the brain. The woman's symptoms include convulsions, and it can be a life-threatening disorder for both mother and baby. Regular antenatal care is the best prevention.

Hydrocephalus
An excessive amount of cerebro-spinal fluid within the skull, leading to an enlarged head, which needs draining. Otherwise it can cause brain damage. The lay term is 'water on the brain'. It often accompanies spina bifida.

Hypoplastic left-heart syndrome
A serious, usually fatal congenital heart disease which affects one or two newborn babies per 10,000 live births. It involves a poorly formed ventricle on the left side of the heart, plus other defects such as a malformed aorta (the heart's main artery). At birth the baby may seem healthy, but within a day or two he or she becomes pale and breathless and usually dies.

Hypospadias
A congenital defect of the penis, where the urethra does not lie in the correct position, so the boy cannot urinate from the end of his penis. In severe cases, the testes are undescended.

Hystero-salpingogram
An X-ray examining the uterus and fallopian tubes.

IVF
In vitro fertilisation is a method of treating infertility whereby an egg is removed from the ovary and fertilised outside the body. It may be used when the woman's fallopian tubes are blocked. The fertilised egg is then implanted in the womb.

Meconium
The thick, sticky substance normally passed by babies a few days after birth. If meconium is passed before birth, this is usually a sign that the baby is in distress. It may then be inhaled by the baby, which can damage the lungs.

Patent ductus arteriosus
A condition in which the blood vessel that enables blood to bypass the lungs in the foetus fails to close after birth. This places strain on the heart and is associated with breathing difficulties. It can often be treated with drugs or surgery.

Placental insufficiency
This unusual condition usually begins to develop between the twenty-fourth and twenty-sixth weeks of pregnancy, but does not tend to become an obvious problem until after the twenty-eighth week. It means that the placenta grows slowly and fails to mature properly, so it is unable to provide adequate nourishment and oxygen for the developing baby. In severe cases, the baby may die in the womb and be stillborn. The commonest causes are pre-eclampsia and smoking, but it may occur for no apparent reason.

Polyhydramnios
Another term for excessive amniotic fluid, which occurs in one in every 250 pregnancies or 10 per cent of multiple births. It can cause premature labour and may indicate foetal abnormality or malformations, especially anencephaly (absence of brain). It may also be called polyhydrama.

Pre-eclampsia
A serious condition, characterised by high blood pressure, oedema (fluid swelling in the tissues) and protein in the urine, which affects about 7 per cent of all pregnancies during the second half of pregnancy. If untreated it can lead to eclampsia. Usually, bed rest and drugs to treat high blood pressure are required; in urgent cases, delivery by emergency Caesarean section may be necessary.

Sonicaid
An instrument commonly used by a midwife to measure foetal heart rate variations and to check foetal wellbeing. Most parents will encounter this at routine antenatal check-ups.

Spina bifida
A congenital defect where one or more vertebrae fail to develop, completely exposing a little of the spinal cord. It is most common in the lower back. The incidence is about 30 babies in every 100,000. Women are now encouraged to take folic acid before

becoming pregnant and early in pregnancy; this is believed to reduce the risk of the defect occurring.

Tentorial tear
A birth injury caused when the baby's head passes along the birth canal. It may happen in pre-term labour because the foetal skull bones are soft, during prolonged labour, as a result of a very rapid delivery or where the baby's head is very large or in an extended position.

Toxaemia
See entry for eclampsia.

Translocation
A rearrangement of the chromosomes inside the cells, a type of mutation. In many cases it causes few problems, but it may lead to a chromosomal abnormality; for example, chromosomes 21 and 14 may join together.

Triple test
Also known as Bart's test this is a blood test offered to many women during pregnancy to assess their statistical risk of carrying a child with certain abnormalities. It measures three substances in the maternal blood: alphafetoprotein, human chorionic gonadotrophin and unconjugated oestriol. A positive result which suggests a high risk usually requires further testing, such as amniocentesis.

Trisomy
The presence of an extra chromosome, so that there are three of a particular number present rather than the usual two. Results range from miscarriage and stillbirth to many physical abnormalities. Trisomy 21 is known as Down's syndrome (see separate entry). Trisomy 18 (Edward's syndrome) and Trisomy 13 (Patau's syndrome) are not common. Children with trisomies other than Down's syndrome usually die early in infancy.

Vernix
The white, greasy substance covering the skin of a newborn baby.

Bibliography

Articles

Sue Alexander, 'Grieving and Caring – A Student Midwife's Perceptions', in *Midwives Chronicle & Nursing Notes*, August 1987.

Born Too Soon, Office of Health Economics, 1993.

Diane Chesterton, 'Stillbirth & the Adolescent', *Modern Midwife*, February 1996.

Pamela Hughes, 'The Management of Bereaved Mothers: What is Best?', in *Midwives Chronicle & Nursing Notes*, August 1987.

Jenni Thomas, 'Maternity Bereavement Counselling: How it has Changed', in *British Journal of Midwifery*, October, 1994, vol. 2, no. 10.

Books

Child Bereavement Trust, *Grieving after the Death of Your Baby*, 1995.

Susan Hill, *Family*, Michael Joseph, 1989.

Nancy Kohner and Alix Henley, *When a Baby Dies – the Experience of Late Miscarriage, Stillbirth & Neonatal Death*, Pandora, 1991.

Jacqueline Vincent Priya, *Birth Traditions & Modern Pregnancy Care*, Element, 1992.

Betty Sweet, *Mayes' Midwifery – A Textbook for Midwives*, 11th edn., Ballière Tindall, 1988.

Marjorie Tew, *Safer Childbirth*, Chapman Hall, 1990.

Jenni Thomas, 'Supporting Parents When Their Baby Dies – A Guide for Professionals', a booklet which accompanies a video, Child Bereavement Trust, 1993.

Statistical Information

Annual Report of the Registrar-General for Northern Ireland, 1994, General Register Office, 1995.

Love, labour and loss

Office of Population Censuses and Surveys, *Infant & Perinatal Mortality, 1994*, Monitor DH3 95/1, Government Statistical Service, 1995 (for statistics on England and Wales).
Scottish Stillbirth and Neonatal Death Report 1994, Information and Statistics Division of the NHS in Scotland, 1995.

Videos

Death at Birth: Miscarriage, Stillbirth, Neonatal Death and Termination for Abnormality, Child Bereavement Trust.
A video aimed at health professionals and trainers.
Empty Arms, Yorskhire Television, 1993.
Available from Yorkshire Television Ltd, Television Centre, Leeds, LS3 1JS.
When Our Baby Died, Child Bereavement Trust.
A video for parents.

Index